C000139429

FOOD SOLUTIONS
Menopause

FOOD SOLUTIONS
Menopause

Recipes & advice to relieve symptoms

Sally Lewis

hamlyn

SAFETY NOTE

This book should not be considered a replacement for professional medical treament. A doctor should be consulted in all matters relating to health, particularly in respect of any symptoms which may require diagnosis or medical attention. While the advice and information in this book are believed to be accurate, neither the author nor the publisher can accept any legal responsibility for any injury or illness sustained while following the treatments and diet plan.

First published in Great Britain in 2001 by
Hamlyn, a division of Octopus Publishing Group Ltd
2–4 Heron Quays, London E14 4JP

This revised edition published 2004

Copyright © Octopus Publishing Group Ltd 2001, 2004

All rights reserved. No part of this work may be reproduced or utilized in any form or by any means, electronic or mechanical, including photocopying, recording or by any information storage and retrieval system, without the prior written permission of the publisher.

ISBN 0 600 61057 8

A CIP catalogue record for this book is available from the British Library

Printed and bound in the United Kingdom by Mackays of Chatham

10 9 8 7 6 5 4 3 2 1

Contents

	Introduction	7
1	The menopause – what is it?	11
2	Your body during the menopause	21
3	Helping yourself	33
4	Orthodox treatment	55
5	Complementary therapies	71
6	The food link	83
7	Recipes	111
	Glossary	225
	General index	229
	Recipe index	233

Introduction

Virtually all women tend to regard the menopause as a time of significant change – physically, psychologically and emotionally – and many dread its onset. Although a woman's body does undergo important changes during and following her menopause, this does not have to be a negative experience. Many women find fresh sources of enjoyment and satisfaction in this new phase of life and are able to manage menopausal symptoms with varying combinations of conventional and complementary treatment in addition to changes to their lifestyle and diet.

In Western societies, which put a high value on youth, the menopause is associated with the ageing process and so all too often is seen as the beginning of an inevitable decline. At one time it was a subject shrouded in secrecy and hedged around with taboos, and even now many people wrongly believe that once a woman's menopause is over, she inevitably becomes wrinkled, dried up and bent. However, in parts of the world where older people are respected and even revered, a post-menopausal woman may be treated quite differently and regarded as a fount of wisdom and useful experience.

Both medical scientists and, equally important, women themselves are now discovering more about the changes that take place around the time of the menopause and how best to handle them. Virtually every week, if not every day, an item appears somewhere in the media about new findings, treatments, diet or other self-help approaches that minimize the ill-effects of the hormonal changes that underlie the menopause. Although they are not the result of any illness, many of the common symptoms associated with the menopause are easier to deal with and alleviate when you understand what is causing them and what you yourself can do about them. The more women understand the changes that are taking place in their bodies, and the possible consequences, the easier it becomes to approach them in a positive and constructive way.

Recognizing and taking steps to alleviate physical symptoms are, however, not always sufficient by themselves. For many women, such physical problems are less significant than the sense that the menopause signals the end of their femininity, their sexual appeal and interest, and that henceforth they will become increasingly 'invisible' to the rest of the world. It can seem as if loss of fertility means that you are no longer a real woman and the best years of your life are over. There is no reason to accept any of these outdated attitudes, and the more positive you are able to be about what you want to do with the rest of your life the better. It is important to realize that your body does not age more rapidly after the menopause and that you can do a great deal to maintain your health and fitness for many years to come. The menopause does not signal the end of your sex life either: many women find that not having to worry about contraception liberates their libido and their enjoyment of sex actually increases. If you see the menopause as the beginning of a new phase in your life rather than as an end, you will improve your enjoyment of the years that follow as much as the ones that went before.

The way the menopause affects you and how you deal with it will be unique to you. Some women have few symptoms or only very minor ones; others may need conventional and/or complementary treatment to alleviate troublesome symptoms. The various forms of complementary therapy not only help with these, but also improve your state of mind, easing tension and lifting your mood. Changes to your lifestyle can enhance your health and sense of wellbeing whether or not you have any symptoms, especially if you make sure you are following the right kind of diet. There is evidence that certain foods improve hormonal balance, as well as contributing to the efficient functioning of your immune system and keeping bodily functions in good working order.

The important thing to bear in mind is that you are in control: you can choose what steps to take and decide which is the right road for you. This book aims to help you make these choices by providing information about all the options available. Whatever you do, you will benefit from thinking about your diet and making adjustments to ensure that you are getting all the nutrients you need. Once you have decided what changes to make, you will find plenty of inspiration in the recipes in this book. Take your pick from the delicious dishes on offer, confident that the meals you make will not only enhance your health but will also taste wonderful too!

1 The menopause – what is it?

For all its unpleasant associations with ageing, loss of femininity and decline, the menopause is an inevitable physical fact of life for every woman who has ever menstruated. For some it is accompanied by major symptoms, for others it is relatively trouble-free. No two women will have identical experiences. Some will find that the process is over and done with quite quickly, but for others it takes years to complete. It can bring emotional trauma or a feeling of liberation and freedom, but in one form or another it is an experience most women will share.

In this chapter you will learn about the hormonal changes that occur during the run up to the menopause, when it is likely to occur, and how to recognize whether you are menopausal.

So what exactly is the menopause?

We tend to use the word menopause rather loosely. Sometimes we mean the extended process of the menstrual cycle beginning to change as hormone levels start declining until periods finally stop; sometimes we mean the point at which a woman has her last ever period. As the word menopause comes from Greek words meaning the cessation of the menses (or monthly periods), we should really use it only if referring to the point in time when a woman has her last period. That is when she can accurately be said to be experiencing the menopause. Of course, in reality that point is identifiable only with hindsight; you will not know your last period is indeed your last until another 12 months or so have passed without another one.

To avoid this kind of confusion, doctors use the word 'climacteric' to include the complete process of hormonal changes from the time when oestrogen levels start to drop, usually well before the actual menopause, to the few years following the last period. Within this process, various different stages are identified by the medical profession.

The various stages

Pre-menopause this term is used in slightly different ways. It may simply mean the whole time your menstrual cycle is running normally until you start to experience the changes which herald the approach of the menopause. Alternatively, it may be used in a narrower sense to refer to the phase when your hormone levels begin to change in the run-up to the menopause, causing changes in your menstrual cycle and the nature of your periods.

Peri-menopause this covers the years either side of your menopause as strictly defined. In other words, it includes the few years before your periods actually stop, when you may begin to get symptoms such as irregular bleeding or hot flushes, and the years after when you have actually had your last period although you do not yet know it for sure.

Menopause your very last period, so this is a diagnosis that can be made only after the event, when you have not had a period for a year.

Post-menopause this refers to the few years immediately after you have actually had your last period and, because of the time lapse needed to be certain this has happened, it overlaps with the peri-menopausal phase and the menopause itself. Once you are post-menopausal you are that way forever.

What causes the climacteric?

To understand what happens to a woman's body during the climacteric we need to start at the very beginning. All baby girls are born with the full complement of eggs they will ever need, stored within their ovaries in an immature state. They start to be released during puberty, ready for possible fertilization following the onset of menstruation.

The menstrual cycle

Like the other hormonal systems within the body, the menstrual cycle is under the ultimate control of a gland in the brain called the hypothalamus, which initiates a cascade of different hormones. It begins when the pituitary gland at the base of the brain, responding to a chemical called gonadotrophin-releasing hormone (GnRh) from the hypothalamus, releases another hormone, FSH, or follicle-stimu-lating hormone. This has the effect of causing one of the egg-containing follicles within an ovary to mature and become fully ripe, at which point the follicle starts to release the female hormone oestrogen (estrogen in the USA). Oestrogen triggers an increase in the blood supply to the uterus, so that its lining thickens and builds up, ready to receive a fertilized egg (or ovum) in due course. Oestrogen levels are normally at their peak just before ovulation and then gradually decline. The hypothalamus and the pituitary gland respond to this high level of oestrogen by secreting smaller quantities of FSH. Once the follicle is fully mature, the pituitary gland secretes another hormone, LH, or luteinizing hormone, to rupture the follicle and set the ovum off on its journey down a Fallopian tube to the uterus. This is what is called ovulation and normally happens around 14 days before the start of the next period.

The empty follicle (which has now developed into the corpus luteum) secretes the female hormone progesterone, which helps to further prepare the woman's body for pregnancy by sensitizing tissue in the breasts, uterine lining and vaginal walls. If the egg is not fertilized within around seven days of ovulation, the follicle dissolves. This results in a drop in progesterone production and this, together with falling oestrogen levels, sets off the shedding of the uterine lining in the form of menstrual flow around two weeks after the egg was originally released from the ovary. The first day of a period is normally regarded as the first day of the menstrual cycle, which is usually around 28 days from beginning to end, although some women have naturally longer or shorter cycles. A cycle ranging in length from 20 up to 36 days may be normal for an individual woman. On around the fifth day of the new cycle, another egg begins to mature and the whole process is repeated, unless an egg is fertilized.

During menstruation, the uterine muscle contracts under the influence of chemicals called prostaglandins, which are responsible for the cramp-like pains which many women experience at the beginning of a period. Sometimes, heavy or painful periods may be the result of an imbalance in the female hormones and the symptoms of premenstrual syndrome (PMS) may also be related to fluctuating levels or unusual sensitivity to such changes, but no one really understands the mechanisms involved.

When changes begin

At some point during a woman's lifetime, the ovaries begin to work less effectively and the levels of oestrogen and progesterone begin to decline. As this happens, you may start to notice changes in your menstrual cycle or experience symptoms related to oestrogen deprivation. The average age for this process of ovarian failure to begin is the mid-forties, and from this point on the rhythmical rise and fall of hormone levels may be disrupted. Two main factors are at work here: fewer follicles develop to maturity and the supply of eggs starts running low, so ovulation may not take place in every cycle.

This has consequences in terms of the normal pattern of changes in hormonal levels throughout the menstrual cycle. If the follicle does not ripen, less oestrogen is produced during the first two weeks of the menstrual cycle. Because there is no mature egg in the follicle, it does not break down to release the egg and form into the corpus luteum. If ovulation doesn't happen, neither does the release of progesterone by the corpus luteum in the second half of the cycle. This means that the oestrogen continues building up the uterine lining without being counterbalanced by the effects of progesterone, and this may result in an unusually heavy period. Ultimately, the failure of the ovaries to release a mature egg on a regular basis will cause oestrogen levels to drop so low that the uterine lining is not stimulated to prepare to accommodate a fertilized egg. To begin with, this may happen in some cycles and not others, so menstruation will not occur every time.

As oestrogen and progesterone levels fall, the hypothalamus and the pituitary gland try to correct the situation by increasing the output of FSH and LH to stimulate the ovaries into normal activity. If the ovaries are not able to respond by developing a follicle to maturity in every cycle, the rising levels of FSH and LH may disrupt the normal operation of other bodily systems, including metabolism, brain chemistry and bone maintenance.

Am I starting my menopause?

Although the average age for a woman to have her menopause is said to be 51, this actually means that half of all women will have it at an earlier age and half when they are over 51. Research in the USA has found that all women will have stopped having periods by the time they reach the age of 58, although the vast majority will have done so four years earlier. It is often said that a woman will have her menopause at about the same age as her mother had hers, although there is no research evidence to support this view. Similarly, the age at which you started your periods may have some bearing on the age at which you stop, but again science has not yet proved this to be the case. Neither motherhood nor the oral contraceptive pill influences the timing of the menopause, but there are several other lifestyle factors which may play a role, generally because they affect oestrogen levels. For example, if you weigh more than about 59kg (9st 4lb), you will have proportionately more fat cells in your body than a lighter woman. Since these cells make oestrogen, the more of them you have, the later your menopause is likely to be. Women who have a medical condition which increases their oestrogen levels, such as diabetes or fibroids, are also likely to continue to menstruate for longer. Eating a healthy diet may also prolong menstruation – under-nourished women tend to have an earlier menopause than those who are well nourished.

A number of factors can increase the likelihood that a woman will start her menopause much earlier than average. For a small proportion of women, ovarian failure can begin in their early thirties (or occasionally even before) without any obvious reason: their internal biological clock seems to be running a little ahead of itself. Smoking can also affect the timing of the menopause: in general, women who smoke tend to stop menstruating at a younger age than those who do not. It is known that female smokers have lower than normal blood levels of oestrogen, although the mechanism involved is not yet well understood by scientists. The majority of women who experience an early menopause do so as a result of surgery to remove their ovaries, usually because of cancer. Radiotherapy treatment for cancer directed at the pelvic region can also damage the ovaries and stop them from working normally. If your ovaries are left in place when you have a hysterectomy (as is often the case), your menopause is likely to begin earlier than it would otherwise have done, although this will be far less sudden and dramatic than if your ovaries are removed at the same time as your uterus. Occasionally, sterilization which involves tying the Fallopian tubes can reduce the blood flow to the ovaries and so accelerate the onset of the menopause.

There are a number of illnesses, mostly those known as auto-immune diseases in which the body's immune system mistakenly attacks its own tissues, which can bring on an early menopause because of damage to the ovaries and the eggs within them. Examples of these include lupus (systemic lupus erythematosus or SLE) and rheumatoid arthritis. Occasionally, the ovaries can be damaged by a bout of mumps, but this is uncommon.

When menstruation ends

Once you have noticed that your menstrual pattern is changing, you can be sure that, sooner or later, you will stop having periods altogether. However, the length of time before this happens varies considerably from one woman to another, as do the number and frequency of your periods and the type of bleeding you will experience in the meantime. The most common pattern is for periods to become lighter and shorter, with the odd one failing to come along when expected. Eventually menstruation tails off completely and you finally realize that you have had your last ever period.

An alternative and also relatively common pattern is for the menstrual cycle to become more unpredictable and inconsistent, with your menstrual flow becoming heavier or lighter or fluctuating between the two. The gaps between periods may become longer or shorter than they used to be, and you may even think it is all over, only to find another period starting after months without one. For a few women, their periods just suddenly stop, without any very noticeable change in the pattern having occurred beforehand, but usually oestrogen levels do not drop sufficiently abruptly for this to happen. A slow and relatively gradual decline is much more common for most women.

Testing for the menopause

Since falling levels of oestrogen are a key factor in the menopause, it might be assumed that measuring the hormone levels in your blood would remove any doubts as to whether you are, in fact, menopausal. In reality, this is not a reliable indication, because levels of oestrogen rise and fall so much over the course of your cycle. However, as we saw on page 16, when oestrogen levels drop as the menopause approaches, the body's 'hormone controller', the hypothalamus, works in conjunction with the pituitary gland to try to restore normal levels by triggering the release of FSH. This hormone stimulates the follicles to ripen so that ovulation will take place. If it is important to know whether you are in fact menopausal, your doctor may arrange a blood test to measure the levels of FSH.

When your periods change it may help to keep a diary so you have a record of what is happening. For example, if your periods are no longer regular, you may experience PMS at odd times and so not recognize it. Record the starting date and duration of each period, the type of bleeding and any symptoms to see what is normal for you. Very long or painful periods or a heavy flow which contains clots could indicate a problem such as fibroids (benign growths in the uterus) and you should report them to your doctor. You should also note if the gaps between periods are less than three weeks, any unexpected bleeding or spotting between periods, especially following sex, or if you have a period after a year or more without one.

2 Your body during the menopause

Before considering the enormous range of symptoms, both physical and psychological, which can be associated with the menopause, it is important to stress that there may be many other factors which could affect a woman's health and mental wellbeing at this period of her life. Friends and family – and even some doctors – may be inclined to ascribe any complaints to the menopause, whether or not they are truly related. The other important point to bear in mind is that the list of symptoms that follows includes everything which might conceivably be related to the hormonal changes surrounding the menopause, even though in reality no one will experience all of them. Indeed, some women will have very few symptoms if any, or the symptoms that they do experience will be only very minor ones.

This chapter describes the range of physical, emotional and psychological symptoms that menopausal women may experience in different degrees and explains what causes them.

Physical symptoms

Hot flushes (or hot flashes or power surges)

These are probably the most common of all menopausal symptoms and may last for several years before and after the final period. How often hot flushes occur and how bad they are will vary from one woman to another; some will have several a day while others may have only one or two a week. The worst of the heat is usually felt across the face, neck and chest, causing a burning sensation as the skin turns red and starts to perspire, sometimes very profusely. A hot flush can last anything from a few minutes to an hour and you will feel your heart beating faster than normal.

Night sweats are the same as hot flushes except that you wake in the night to find yourself drenched in sweat – you may need to change not only your nightclothes but your bedding as well. If this happens regularly, so you rarely get an unbroken night's sleep, you are liable to end up feeling tired and irritable.

Both these problems are a response to fluctuating hormone levels. Alterations in oestrogen levels seem to reduce the body's ability to cool itself through sweating and its natural 'comfort temperature' can become lower as the hypothalamus adjusts the 'thermostat' downwards. The two factors combined can cause the symptoms of a hot flush as the body tries to shed excess heat quickly: blood vessels near the skin dilate, especially around the face, neck and upper body, and the sweat glands go into overdrive.

Genital problems

Falling levels of oestrogen can affect the walls of the vagina and urinary tract, making them thinner and drier, and may also weaken the sphincter muscle which controls the flow of urine out of the bladder. The bladder walls become more sensitive and the need to urinate more frequent, and some women find that urine leaks occasionally when they cough or laugh. This problem, called stress incontinence, is the result of increased pressure inside the abdomen causing drops of urine to be squeezed out past the weakened sphincter.

It is possible for a lack of lubrication in the vagina to make sex uncomfortable or even painful, and infections become more likely because hormonal changes make vaginal secretions more acidic and thus less hostile to many bacteria. Urinary infections may be more common for similar reasons. Overall, the genital area may be itchy and uncomfortable or even sore at times.

Headaches

Women who have always been prone to headaches or who are migraine sufferers may find that the problem becomes worse as they approach the menopause. Specifically, attacks may be more frequent or severe in the week before a period is due to start. This increase in frequency and severity of headaches should diminish once the menopause is complete and the hormonal fluctuations subside. As migraine sufferers know only too well, in addition to a very severe headache an attack often involves other symptoms, which may include visual disturbances, fatigue, nausea and vomiting. However, it is important to remember that headaches can have a wide range of causes which may have nothing to do with the menopause, so if you start to have more headaches or they are much worse than usual, it is worth reporting your symptoms to your doctor.

Breast problems

Many women will be used to the fact that their breasts become tender or lumpy in the week before their period is due, but such symptoms often get worse as the menopause approaches. Breast pain (mastalgia) may occur at the normal time or at any time during the cycle and can be quite debilitating in severe cases. It is thought to be caused by increased sensitivity to fluctuating hormone levels, although the mechanism involved is not as yet fully understood.

Breast cancer is probably top of the list of diseases that women fear and it is a fact that the risk of developing it increases with age. While research is rapidly advancing our understanding of this condition and its causes are not yet completely understood. Many factors have been implicated, including diet – especially saturated fats and alcohol, emotional trauma, exposure to various kinds of pollution and pesticides, and even the changing hormones during the menopause.

It is now known that a minority of women inherit certain genes (known as BRCA1 and BRCA2) that greatly increase the chances of developing breast cancer; such women usually have close female relatives who developed breast cancer before the age of 50. The relationship between oestrogen and the risk of cancer in the breast, cervix, ovaries and endometrium is still under investigation. Other factors that increase the risk of breast cancer are listed on the right.

RISKS FOR BREAST CANCER

○ Early onset of menstruation, late menopause, late pregnancies and never having been pregnant – these all increase the length of time over which the breast is subjected to the influence of oestrogen, progesterone and other hormones produced by the ovary.

○ Weight – obesity is associated with increased risk of breast cancer after the menopause (although not before).

○ Smoking – increases the rate of calcium loss and hastens the onset of osteoporosis.

○ Alcohol – too high an intake can increase the incidence.

○ Benign breast disease – this carries a slight risk depending upon the degree of breast change. Breast lumps that show abnormal cell changes carry a much higher risk.

○ High birth weight – mothers whose babies weighed over 4kg (approximately 9lb) at birth have a higher risk.

○ Diet – Japanese women, whose diet is rich in unsaturated fats, have a lower incidence of breast cancer than Western women, who eat more saturated fat. It was thought that high soya consumption in Japan might also have a protective effect, but recent research has seriously questioned this view.

Joint pains

Muscles and joints may become stiff and painful as hormonal changes cause them to lose some of their strength and elasticity. As well as the lower back, the wrists, knees and ankles tend to be the main problem areas as far as pain is concerned. Again, there may be other reasons for such symptoms and you should talk to your doctor if you experience pain that is more than trivial or short-term.

Skin

Like other tissues elsewhere in the body, the skin will react to the decline in oestrogen. It becomes thinner, less taut and elastic, and wrinkles start to look more noticeable. Usually it becomes drier, blood vessels beneath its surface are more obvious and visible, and bruising occurs more easily. Some women develop patches of brown pigmentation or find their skin is increasingly itchy. In some cases, this may be a sign of a condition known as formication, so called because it feels like ants (*formicae* in Latin) crawling over the skin. Its exact cause is not known, but it usually disappears without treatment eventually.

COLLAGEN AND ELASTIN

These are proteins which make up the connective tissue throughout the body, providing strength and elasticity in joints, muscles and skin, and the tough fibres which hold organs and joints in place. However, the cells that generate these proteins are sensitive to oestrogen and become less active and effective as the level drops. The resultant effects on collagen and elastin fibres can have repercussions throughout the body.

Nails

Finger- and toenails become brittle and split or break easily; some women develop noticeable white spots on their nails.

Hair

The decline in oestrogen slows down the growth rate of hair, which will tend to become thinner, drier and more fragile. Most women notice that their hair gradually loses its former shine and bounce and some develop dandruff for the first time.

Mouth and gums

Some people are bothered by cracking skin at the corners of the mouth and by frequent mouth ulcers that heal very slowly. The mouth sometimes feels uncomfortably dry and the gums get soft and puffy. If the gums start to bleed, infection can become a real problem for both gums and, eventually, teeth.

Masculinization

As oestrogen declines, the effects of androgens become more pronounced. All women produce these male hormones as well as the female ones, but androgen production continues even once the ovaries have stopped secreting oestrogen. Relatively high levels of male hormones encourage the growth of hair on the face and sometimes elsewhere on the upper body and can also result in the voice getting deeper.

Weight gain

Almost all women gain weight after the menopause and find that their shape alters as the fat settles in different places. These are natural consequences of lower oestrogen levels and a tendency for the metabolism – the rate at which the body consumes 'fuel' – to slow as you get older. However, there is something to be said in favour of a little extra weight: although your ovaries stop secreting oestrogen the fat cells continue to do so, so carrying a little extra fat – say 4.5kg (10lb) – will increase your oestrogen level and help to counter the effects of its decline.

Prolapse

In some women, the weakening of the fibres in the soft tissue holding various internal organs (such as the uterus, bladder, urethra and rectum) in place may cause them to drop. Such problems usually affect women whose internal supports have been weakened as a result of giving birth.

Osteoporosis

This is a serious condition that affects mainly post-menopausal women and means that bones break easily after minor falls or stresses; it can also result in the upper spine becoming deformed into a 'dowager's hump'. In healthy people, bone is lost and replaced on a regular basis, the whole process under the control of hormones, including oestrogen. As hormone levels decline, bone is not replaced as quickly and the result is a weakening of the bones. Spaces develop within the bones, giving them a sponge-like appearance and making them more brittle.

Most at risk are small, slim women whose bone mass is lower than average, poorly nourished women, heavy smokers, women with medical conditions such as rheumatoid arthritis, amenorrhoea (absence of periods) or an over-active thyroid, and those on medical treatments such as steroid drugs. In addition, women who have never taken much exercise of the weight-bearing kind and those whose diet has been low in calcium are at increased risk of osteoporosis. Since oestrogen is important in efficient bone replacement, women who have had an early menopause, a hysterectomy together with removal of the ovaries, or surgical removal of the ovaries may also lose bone mass at a more rapid rate and an earlier age than they might otherwise do. Research is currently under way to determine what role may be played by genetic factors in determining who will develop osteoporosis, but, this apart, it could be said that your level of risk is a reflection of the life you have lived for the previous 20 to 30 years.

Black women (because they usually reach a higher peak bone mass than white women) and those who have had several pregnancies (conception is accompanied by an oestrogen surge) face a lower risk of developing osteoporosis. Although bone loss begins to decline from the age of around 35, it does not normally drop low enough to result in osteoporosis for some years after the menopause. Thus the older you are, the greater your risk.

Cardiovascular disease

Prior to the decline in oestrogen levels which begins in the years running up to the cessation of menstruation, women are partially protected by oestrogen from the risk of problems affecting the blood vessels and the heart itself. There is an increased tendency with age for the coronary arteries to become 'furred up' (much like the inside of a kettle) as patches of plaque accumulate on the inner surfaces. Plaque is a fatty substance made up of atheroma, which projects from the smooth artery walls, narrowing the channel through which blood travels and interfering with normal flow. Clots may form on the artery walls and if one breaks off it may move away from its point of origin and lodge in a smaller vessel, blocking the flow completely.

If the blood supply to the heart becomes impeded, the result will be angina or, in extreme cases, a heart attack. Chest pains that occur following quite minor exertion, and sometimes stress or emotional upset, are the main symptom of angina, which can usually be treated by drugs or, if necessary, by surgery. Although men are much more vulnerable to cardiovascular disease from their forties, by the age of 55 or so both sexes face a similar risk.

Stroke

Although stroke is generally more common in older people, changes resulting from the menopause are not thought to be a specific risk factor, although high oestrogen levels may offer a small degree of protection.

Psychological and emotional problems

As scientists' understanding of the brain expands, it is becoming clear that there is a close link between the body and the mind. In particular, the discovery of oestrogen receptors in various parts of the brain has revealed that the hormone plays an important role in controlling many functions, including memory, perception and especially mood. This explains why women complain of memory loss and forgetfulness as their oestrogen levels go into decline at the menopause. It may also be responsible for creating that sense of anxiety – unrelated to life events or problems – that troubles so many menopausal women. Oestrogen receptors in a region of the brain called the amygdala seem to respond to the hormone by creating a general sense of wellbeing and by increasing interest in sex, so when levels of oestrogen drop, these aspects are inevitably adversely affected.

The brain also has receptors for the other major female hormone, progesterone, and these appear to be related to mood. High levels of the hormone can trigger depression in susceptible women, which may account for the low mood which often develops in the premenstrual week. Women who respond to progesterone sometimes have similar symptoms when taking combined hormone replacement therapy (HRT, see page 65). Emotional symptoms are thus linked to premenstrual symptoms where hormone levels fluctuate. Emotional symptoms can be disabling and are often, though not inevitably, the result of fluctuating hormone levels.

Many emotional problems have psychological origins, but you should consider whether they could be caused by other factors in your life. At this time, children will have left the home and parents may be ageing and bring new responsibilities. Divorce, bereavement and financial strains all bring great changes, and symptoms such as depression can be dismissed as menopausal when they are not. In countries where older women are respected for their wisdom, their psychological, emotional and physical symptoms are reputed to be much lower. If you are able to be positive and make up your mind that you will readjust and rediscover yourself, you will find that you can approach the menopause in a more positive frame of mind.

Once you decide to take responsibility for your own wellbeing, there are many treatments available, both orthodox and complementary, plus changes you can make to your lifestyle and eating habits. All of these will increase your chances of a trouble-free menopause. Remember that while there may be many symptoms associated with the menopause, you will not necessarily experience them all, or any at all, in a severe form.

Emotional symptoms

- ❏ Anxiety
- ☒ Depression
- ❏ Fear of ageing
- ❏ Feeling unable to cope
- ☒ Forgetfulness
- ❏ Irritability
- ☒ Lack of concentration
- ❏ Lack of energy and motivation
- ☒ Lack of self-confidence
- ❏ Lack of self-esteem
- ❏ Loss of sex drive
- ❏ Mood swings
- ☒ Tearfulness
- ❏ Vulnerability

3 Helping yourself

For many women, the prospect of the oncoming menopause is extremely daunting, if not depressing. Fear of the impending physical and emotional changes and not knowing what to expect are often exacerbated by gloomy or alarming stories in the media. Yet there may be no need to anticipate the menopause with trepidation. Change is part of life and something everyone has to face at particular points, whether it is through choice or circumstance or a combination of both these things.

The menopause can, if you let it, be turned into an opportunity for reflection and awareness. You will benefit from finding time to look back on what you have achieved so far and to think about what you want in the future and how you plan to make the most of life from now on. By focusing on yourself and your future, you make it possible to take responsibility for what happens in your life, to be open to new and enjoyable experiences.

A positive approach

Many women today will live a third of their total life-span after the menopause – an experience that was comparatively rare in earlier generations. We all know that our bodies change as we get older, but for most women the menopause begins around the same time that they start to notice visible signs of ageing. Yet this does not automatically imply that you will be in need of medical attention. Many women go through the menopause with few or no serious symptoms or problems, although some of course may have more than their fair share of troubles. Your approach to this new stage of your life will have an important influence on how you deal with the changes that are taking place in your body. A positive outlook, an ability to adapt and making time to take a fresh look at your lifestyle will all help you to cope. Some changes are likely to be beyond your control, such as children leaving home or changes in your role at work or your responsibilities towards ageing parents, and you may well wonder what you should do for the best. Taking steps to make sure you remain as healthy as possible and looking after your own emotional and psychological wellbeing will improve your chances of handling whatever should come along in this next phase of your life.

A good social life

If family life with your partner and children has been the mainstay of your life up to now, you can easily feel isolated and bereft when the time comes for your offspring to move away.

Some women feel a sense of loss when the cessation of their periods means they have to accept that children are no longer even a theoretical possibility; others are simply thankful that contraception is no longer important. Natural concerns about ageing and the increased risk of health problems such as osteoporosis and heart disease can, to a considerable extent, be alleviated by following the advice in this book. Depression can sometimes accompany the menopause, but, as well as seeking any treatment that is necessary, making sure you have a good social network can do much to keep it at bay.

It is important to have friends with whom you can share the bad times as well as the good. Having friends who encourage you to join in social activities can help you to feel positive about yourself and keep up vital links with the outside world. Those women who do experience troublesome menopausal symptoms often find them more manageable if they can share their experiences with others who are going or have gone through something similar.

Many women find that changing home circumstances mean they now have more time and energy to take up new activities and join groups where they make new friends. Plenty of organizations now target those aged over 50, but even if you are not sure whether these are for you, the option is always there and may be worth exploring. Try not to rule out any possibilities, especially if you have previously been very much involved in family life and have had little incentive or opportunity to develop separate personal friendships and activities up until now. This can be a good time to follow up an interest you have always had but for which you have never previously had time or energy to spare. Many women find that they enter a new, creative phase of life after the menopause and develop hitherto unexplored talents in spheres such as writing, painting, the decorative arts or dance, for example.

The opportunity to put yourself and your personal needs first can be a new and very rewarding experience. Wherever you happen to live, you will surely find many activities on offer, some of which will be right for you. There are classes in just about everything you can think of, as well as books, cassettes and videos that can introduce you to a whole range of intriguing possibilities. In the following pages, you will find some suggestions which can serve as a starting point while you consider all the possible options. In particular, you might think of exploring some relaxation techniques and yoga, which have much to offer in terms of improved mental and physical wellbeing and easing minor menopausal symptoms.

Relaxation techniques

Many women who practise relaxation sessions on a daily basis have found that these help to ease hot flushes. With some claiming a reduction in symptoms of up to half, it really is worth finding the time to try the techniques for yourself. Contrary to a commonly held belief, there is much more to relaxation than simply sitting in a comfortable chair with a magazine or watching TV. The techniques have to be learned and practised, and although some master them relatively easily, others find it takes time to learn how to do so. Fortunately, there is a lot of help available: you can buy cassette and video tapes if you prefer to learn at home or you can join a class, where you will also have the opportunity to meet new people and an incentive to attend on a regular basis.

One of the most important benefits of learning how to relax properly is that you can use the techniques to counter the ill-effects of stress. Despite its bad reputation, stress does have some positive aspects, as it helps to galvanize us into taking necessary action when required, but too much or constant stress can deplete the body's resources and have a detrimental effect on health. When you are feeling completely stressed out and about to explode, trying to make yourself relax can be a real challenge. However, once you have mastered the techniques you will be aware of when you are experiencing stress and so be better able to deal with it before it gets out of hand. Developing an awareness of your body and the signals it sends out makes stressful situations much easier to deal with. Relaxation techniques have the effect of slowing a rapid heartbeat, regulating breathing and controlling the metabolic rate. They also reduce your adrenaline levels, which rise when you are under stress, allow the immune system to function more effectively and can ease related symptoms such as headaches and migraines.

Simple relaxation   there are many different techniques but one simple tried and tested method is consciously to tense and relax every muscle in the body in turn. When practising this technique, make sure that you choose a quiet room where you will not be disturbed; if necessary take the phone off the hook and disconnect the door bell.

1 Lie or sit comfortably, close your eyes and become aware of your body. Try not to think about any worries or tasks that need doing and concentrate your attention on your body and, in particular, on any areas of physical tension.

2 Breathe in deeply and slowly through your nose, then exhale slowly through your mouth.

3 Allow your tongue to come away from the roof of your mouth and relax the lips and surrounding muscles as you continue to breathe in and out.

4 Focus on your feet, tightening your toes as you inhale, then hold for a count of five. Exhale through your mouth, releasing your toes.

5 Now work up through your body, tightening each set of muscles in turn, starting with your calves, then releasing them after a count of five.

6 Continue to tense and release each major set of muscles until you have worked on those in your neck and face.

7 Now continue to breathe deeply and slowly for a few minutes before opening your eyes and stretching your whole body. You should feel relaxed and refreshed.

Visualization

An alternative name for this technique is 'creative imagery', because it involves summoning up mental images that encourage a sense of relaxation and tranquillity. Positive visualization can be associated with achieving a specific goal – which is why competitive athletes often use it as part of their mental preparation and motivational training. Even if youhave no interest in scoring goals or breaking sprint records, you can use the same method to help you overcome particular worries and fears.

Before you begin, select an image that is associated in your mind with calm and relaxation such as a beautiful sunset or a peaceful beach or country scene.

Simple visualization choose a quiet, comfortable location where you will not be disturbed and find a comfortable place to sit or lie down.

1 Close your eyes and breathe slowly and deeply in through your nose and out through your mouth.

2 Try to create an image of your chosen scene in your mind and hold it there.

3 Use your other senses to fill in the picture: smell the flowers in the garden, for example, or listen to the sound of the waves on the shore.

4 Keep your breathing regular and relaxed, pushing aside any intrusive thoughts, concentrating only on the mental image you have chosen.

5 Stay in this place as long as you like, then gently bring yourself back to the present. Imagine yourself leaving the scene slowly and coming back to reality, then open your eyes, giving yourself time to readjust.

Meditation

This is similar to relaxation and is another way of freeing your mind from distressing or worrying thoughts. The main difference is that it uses a sound or short phrase as a mental focus point to clear away intrusive thoughts. With practice, meditation can achieve a very deep level of relaxation. There is some evidence that daily meditation can help to lower raised blood pressure and ease headaches, migraine symptoms and other stress-related problems. There are many different approaches to meditation and the technique is best learned from a teacher or by following the instructions on a cassette, but you can try at home by selecting your word or phrase, then focusing on it in the same way as in the visualization technique above. Instead of conjuring the image, you simply repeat the words (or mantra) whenever unwanted thoughts intrude.

Yoga

You don't have to be a contortionist or even particularly supple to learn simple yoga, and everyone can benefit from practising this ancient Eastern art. If possible, you should learn from a qualified teacher, as it is difficult to know whether you are doing the movements correctly on your own. It is easy to find beginners' classes almost everywhere and experienced teachers encourage everyone to work at their own pace. Yoga offers both physical and mental benefits: it stretches the body and clears the mind, promoting a sense of calm and peace. As you become more proficient, you will find that your body becomes stronger and more flexible and you cope more easily with mental stress. Most beginners' classes in the West concentrate on Hatha yoga, which involves practising breathing (*pranayama*), poses (*asanas*) and meditation (*dhyana*). The breathing exercises are important because they improve physical energy and vitality as well as toning the circulation and strengthening the lungs. Yoga is beneficial for women of menopausal age because you work at your own pace, progressing to the more difficult moves without placing undue stress on your body. It can help to ease symptoms such as headaches, hot flushes, depression and anxiety and improves overall muscular tone and flexibility.

The Alexander technique

This is a way of re-educating the body out of bad habits of movement and posture that have been acquired over the years.

Originally developed by Frederick Alexander, it involves using a combination of gentle instruction and guided movement which is designed to help you to rediscover your natural physical poise, grace and freedom of movement and so eliminate postural strains and symptoms such as pain and tension arising from them. It is possible to learn the basics from a book or a video, but it is far better to attend classes with a teacher who can tailor the techniques to your personal needs and ensure that you are moving correctly.

Exercise

The very word is enough to elicit a groan from people who have done virtually no exercise for years and find even thinking about the prospect daunting if not exhausting. Yet the benefits are very real and can hardly be over-stressed. This is particularly true for women around the time of the menopause, because taking the right kind of exercise not only boosts general health but is also very effective in controlling weight gain, lifting depression, relieving anxiety, alleviating insomnia and improving self-esteem.

Weight-bearing exercise is especially important in this phase of your life, because it helps to strengthen bones and stave off osteoporosis (see page 28). Walking, jogging, racket sports, dancing, aerobics, skating and skipping all qualify as weight-bearing and it is literally never too late to begin and gain the benefits. As well as increasing your energy and vitality, exercise is great for lifting your mood and keeping depression at bay. In purely physical terms, regular exercise that works up a light sweat and leaves you breathing a little faster than usual will tone up your whole cardiovascular system, leaving you less vulnerable to diseases that affect your heart, blood vessels and lungs, as well as firming your muscles and other soft tissue.

When you have been exercising on a regular basis for just a few weeks, you will notice that you are able to cope better with stress, and your improved fitness and sense of wellbeing will give you an enormous lift. Some of the psychological benefits of regular exercise are thought to be due to the fact that it stimulates the production of brain chemicals called endorphins, sometimes known as 'feel-good chemicals'. These create a feeling of calm and alertness and are very effective at countering any tendency to low moods.

Other hormones stimulated by exercise can actually have the effect of making you feel less hungry than you might expect afterwards, and many people say they feel less tempted by 'unhealthy' foods like sweet and fatty fare. In fact, the best fuel for exercise is complex carbohydrates such as pasta, which release a steady supply of energy in the form of blood glucose. They are also the best way to top up your energy levels afterwards. Make sure to replace lost fluids by drinking plenty of water both during and after strenuous exercise.

The trouble with exercise is that you can't store it up – you have to keep on doing it or the benefits will be lost before very long. However, the good news is that once you have felt and seen those benefits for yourself, you won't want to stop, even if you have been a couch potato all your life up until now.

Bone health

The main reason why weight-bearing exercise is so vital is, as we have seen, the role it plays in improving bone density and so lessening the risk of osteoporosis developing following the menopause. In fact, the earlier in life you begin taking this type of exercise, the greater the beneficial effects, as it will boost the peak bone density, which is usually reached around the age of 35. Earlier generations of women rarely needed to make any deliberate effort to exercise because physical activity was a normal part of their lives: they walked, sometimes long distances, to school, work and the shops, often carrying heavy bags, and probably did hard physical labour in the kitchen and garden as well. Today, when most people normally travel by car or public transport rather than walking and have access to all kinds of labour-saving devices at home, we have to make a special effort to build exercise into our lives unless we are naturally sporty types.

By placing physical stress on our bodies through exercise, we not only encourage the process of building bone but also increase the amount of 'pull' exerted on bones by the muscles attached to them, so further encouraging bone health by making bone-building cells more active. The loss of oestrogen following the menopause accelerates natural bone loss, which begins slowly in the late thirties, so that by the time women reach their mid-sixties, many of them are increasingly vulnerable to fractures because their bones have lost so much of their former strength.

Before we consider specific types of exercise, it is worth bearing in mind that even small increases in physical activity can help: walking rather than driving to the shops or to work, using stairs rather than lifts or escalators, or just giving the dog a slightly longer walk each day. If you have never gone in for exercise, you might start by taking a short but brisk daily walk, increasing your speed and distance as your fitness improves.

You should also check with your doctor before you take up exercise in earnest to see whether there is any activity you should avoid because of existing health problems, or indeed any type which would be particularly beneficial.

Although you need to think about taking exercise for health reasons, you are unlikely to stick with it for long unless you choose an activity you enjoy. If cost is a factor in your decision, think about something that involves relatively little expense, such as walking or jogging, although you will need to invest in the right footwear. You do not need expensive, high-fashion trainers but you do need shoes designed to protect your feet and knees by cushioning the impact with the ground; your nearest sports equipment shops should be able to advise you if necessary. Some people find that paying out for membership of a gym or sports centre gives them the incentive they need to go regularly, and although the initial outlay can be quite high, the cost per visit often works out to be quite reasonable if you use the facilities several times a week. Whatever you choose, aim to build up to five sessions per week of around 30 minutes each; you can do the same thing every time or opt for a mix of different activities to gain maximum benefits.

The aims of exercise

Basically, you need to consider three aspects of fitness: increasing strength, stamina and flexibility.

Strength this does not mean developing muscles like Miss Universe; in fact, to do so is not easy and requires a specific training programme. Becoming strong is something entirely different and, in the majority of cases, means paying particular attention to your upper body. Building up strength in this area will not only improve your posture but will also make many everyday tasks much easier – for example, lifting and carrying heavy items, gardening and decorating will all feel much less of an effort.

Stamina this term actually refers to the amount of oxygen supplied to your muscles by the action of your heart and lungs. When you are unfit, you will find yourself breathless and tired after a short burst of effort such as running for a bus or swimming one length of a pool. You will take a while to recover afterwards and you may just assume this is inevitable as you get older, but that is not the case. You can improve your stamina at any age by taking the kind of exercise that develops the heart and lungs. This means aerobic work: in other words, activity that involves increased uptake of oxygen, such as running, jogging or dancing. Once you have begun exercising, your stamina will increase relatively quickly. Even people who have had a heart attack can recover sufficiently to run a marathon, although, of course, this isn't a suitable or even desirable goal for most people. Walking and jogging cost nothing and can be done in the open air in the right climate, but wherever you are there are likely to be exercise classes of various types or a gym within easy reach.

Flexibility this does not mean the ability to do the splits or move like a ballet dancer. Rather it is about keeping the joints mobile and moving freely, and countering any tendency to stiffness that comes with increasing years. Exercise keeps the muscles around joints strong and flexible and also reduces vulnerability to injury when you happen to move suddenly or awkwardly. Anyone can do daily stretching exercises at home or, if you prefer to join a class, consider taking up yoga, tai chi, chi kung or pilates, which are gentle but very effective.

Take your pick

The best exercise is something you enjoy and so will continue to do on a regular basis. Try to include some of the following weight-bearing types, but the most important thing is to make a start.

Walking much under-estimated as a form of exercise, it is easy and free. All you have to do is rouse yourself to go out and walk briskly for at least 30 minutes. Aim to go fast enough to be slightly out of breath but still able to hold a conversation; any slower and you will not be making any beneficial impact on your heart and lungs.

Jogging start slowly if you have never done it before and do a few minutes' stretching prior to setting off (and again afterwards) to prevent the build-up of lactic acid, which will otherwise leave you with sore muscles. You could begin by alternating walking with jogging until you get a bit fitter. It will alleviate the boredom and encourage you to continue if you can persuade someone else to join you.

Rebounder most sports shops stock these mini-trampolines, which are especially useful if the weather discourages outdoor exercise. Bouncing works your heart and lungs without causing any stress on joints in the lower limbs.

Aerobics you should have no trouble finding a local class, but make sure that the teacher is qualified and avoid anyone who adopts a 'no gain without pain' approach. If you're unfit, go for low-impact aerobics, which is less physically demanding than the high-impact kind. Alternatively, you can choose one of the many aerobics videos to follow at home.

Tai chi this stylized system of movements, which originated in China, requires concentration and controlled breathing. The movements are slow and subtle and are designed to coordinate body, mind and spirit, so they can be good for reducing stress and encouraging relaxation.

Yoga this is very useful for improving overall strength and flexibility through postures and stretching, and most classes involve elements of relaxation and controlled breathing. Good for newcomers to exercise, although advanced yoga is physically demanding.

Pilates a system of coordinated exercise and breathing that is especially good for toning muscles and improving posture while encouraging mental and spiritual calm and harmony.

A healthy sex life

There are many reasons why your sex life may go off the boil around the time of the menopause but it is certainly not inevitable. Plenty of couples continue to have a good physical relationship into their seventies and beyond, so you should not assume that if yours is disappointing there is nothing to be done. The decline may relate to a loss of libido, physical pain or discomfort, problems within your relationship, a loss of confidence in your own sexual attractiveness or even simple boredom – alone or in combination.

Loss of libido can be a consequence of declining oestrogen or sometimes because sexual intercourse is uncomfortable or painful because of vaginal dryness and lack of lubrication. HRT will help with both, and a lubricating jelly will help with dryness. Exercise that tones up the circulation will increase the blood supply to the genital area and you should also make sure your diet includes an adequate supply of vitamins and minerals to keep the tissues healthy and maintain your energy levels. Pelvic floor exercises (see below) will help tighten the vagina if practised frequently and regularly.

If you are concerned about the changes affecting you both mentally and physically around the time of your menopause, try to be as open as you can with your partner about what is

---

SIMPLE PELVIC EXERCISES

○ Each time you go to the loo, try stopping the urine flow midstream; the muscles you use to do this are your pelvic floor muscles.

○ When you have stopped the flow, hold this position for a count of three before releasing the flow.

○ Once you can do this, practise drawing up these muscles at other times, hold for a count of five, then release slowly.

○ Do this exercise whenever you think of it, but no fewer than ten times every day.

---

happening and how you feel. Changing when and where you make love may revive your interest if sex has become too much of a routine. There is no reason why you should have sex only at night in the bedroom, even if that is what you have always done previously. When intercourse does not appeal, see whether your partner would be willing to try a massage session using aromatherapy oils; this can be very relaxing and a nice way of showing your love even when you don't feel like sex. If both of you like the idea of trying something a little different, you could consider creating a special atmosphere with candles, soft music, champagne in bed or even something more outrageous... Remember, you don't have to be serious and if things don't quite work at least you can laugh together.

Sex is good for you. It is relaxing, it releases hormones that lift your mood and it helps sustain a feeling of closeness with your partner. While HRT is often effective at treating problems such as loss of libido, taking it can sometimes create the impression that the menopause is an illness and thus undermine a woman's confidence in her sexuality. In fact, many women find that their interest in sex increases after the menopause: they no longer worry about contraception or being interrupted by the children and have more time and energy. Although oestrogen levels decline, the relative increase in levels of the male hormone testosterone can result in an increased sex drive. Of course, a man may also have difficulties with sex for either physical or psychological reasons. Being open with one another is a good first step, and if necessary, a woman may need to encourage her partner to consult his doctor about a problem such as erectile dysfunction, as this can often be treated effectively.

Caring for your body
Your breasts

All women should develop breast awareness and become familiar with the way their breasts look and feel. This makes it more likely that you will notice any changes and get them professionally checked early on. Most women have strong feelings about their breasts – whether they love or hate them – and these feelings are usually an important element in the way they see themselves and their self-esteem. Few women have breasts that are exactly the same size and shape as one another, and many feel that their breasts are too large or too small. Apart from surgery, however, there is little that can be done to change this. Breasts have no muscle, but the pectoral muscles underneath can be strengthened and developed by exercise so as to provide better support. Breasts are supplied by blood from the major arteries that also supply the chest wall; they are drained through a network of veins.

During the menopause breasts can shrink or become slack as the oestrogen that stimulates the tissues declines and the breast tissue becomes less dense. Some women, on the other hand, find their breasts get bigger as the number of fat cells increases in response to hormonal changes.

It is advisable to examine your breasts monthly, preferably during the week after your period has ended if you are still menstruating. Lumps and bumps are quite common in the week before menstruation, although they tend to disappear after the menopause as oestrogen is no longer stimulating the milk ducts in preparation for pregnancy and birth.

1 Stand facing the mirror, arms by your side, undressed to the waist. Look at your breasts and note any visible change. If you are looking at them for the first time, just take note of the way they look so you can compare it to next time.

2 Raise both arms behind your head, look at your breasts, then do the same thing again turning first to one side and then to the other.

3 Turn to face the mirror, place both hands on your hips and push hard. This should tighten your chest muscles. Note the shape of each breast from every angle.

4 With a soapy hand, in the bath or shower, pass the flat of your fingers all over each breast without squeezing or prodding, using the right hand for the left breast and vice versa. Remember to include the 'tail' of each breast that runs into the armpit and the area below the collarbone. Look for any lumpiness; any dent or dimple in the skin when you lift the arm; any change in skin colour or texture; an inverted nipple; or any discharge or bleeding. Look for any other changes; be aware of what is normal for you.

Your skin

Skin gradually loses elasticity around the menopause and over subsequent years due to declining oestrogen levels, and this is often most obvious on the face. You develop wrinkles and your skin is likely to become much drier. Using moisturizer every day will help but it cannot prevent the underlying changes. The skin also loses its tone because the supporting tissues weaken once your oestrogen levels drop (see Collagen and elastin, page 26). You may also notice small 'liver spots' or moles appearing.

HRT prevents these changes and many women see an improvement in their skin after taking it for a relatively short time. You can slow the progress of this deterioration somewhat by good skin care – especially thorough cleansing, frequent moisturizing, drinking plenty of water and protecting your skin from damaging ultraviolet sunlight. Cover up as much as possible and always use sun-protection preparations, even on cloudy days. Beauty treatments such as facials, massage, face masks, electro-desiccation and chemical skin-peeling can improve the appearance of the skin, although they will not affect the underlying processes responsible for causing the changes. Smoking makes wrinkles worse and alcohol can cause broken blood vessels on the face; on the other hand, a healthy diet rich in vitamins and minerals will help nourish the skin.

Simple facial exercises

Spend a minute on each exercise, practising in front of a mirror to begin with.

Eyes to tone the surrounding muscles and slow down the appearance of crow's feet:

1 Stare hard but with your eyes closed; you will feel tension in the surrounding area.
2 Keeping your eyes shut, tighten them, screwing up and 'looking' inward with your eyes crossed. Hold for a few seconds.
3 Open your eyes as wide as you can and stare at a fixed point.
4 Blink rapidly ten to fifteen times, then close your eyes until you feel that the pupils have returned to normal.

Laughter lines to ease lines running from the outer edge of the nostrils to the corners of the mouth:

1 Raise the corners of your mouth and upper lip, stretching the top lip up and over the teeth while opening your mouth about 2cm. Keep your mouth and neck muscles relaxed, but feel the tension in your cheek pads.

2 Suck the air into one cheek, then move it to the opposite one. Suck the air into both cheeks and the area above your top lip. 'Chew' the air. Repeat five to ten times.

3 Pursing the lips gently, open them about 1cm, as if blowing bubbles, and exhale gently.

Frown lines to tone the muscles that create the vertical lines between your eyebrows:

1 Frown hard, then relax the muscles.

2 Put your three middle fingers from each hand on the outer edge of each eyebrow and frown. Feel the pull on your fingers.

3 Close your eyes and relax the muscles by vibrating your fingertips lightly over your forehead.

4 Orthodox treatment

Like the menstrual cycle and pregnancy, the menopause is neither an illness nor a sign of ill-health, yet it is frequently accompanied by unpleasant symptoms, some of which can be quite disabling. The decision as to whether to seek treatment to alleviate symptoms is one only the individual woman can make. It will depend on a combination of factors, such as her attitude to taking medication, how well she copes without it and how incapacitating her symptoms are. At least if she does choose to consult a doctor, she can be reasonably confident that, unlike in the past, her concerns will be taken seriously and she will be told about the wide range of possible treatments on offer.

Since the symptoms are generally the result of declining levels of the female hormones, the most logical way to alleviate them would seem to be by replacing what's missing: in other words, to take some form of HRT. This will be the appropriate treatment for many women, but it is not the only option. Other treatments can be given to tackle specific problems, such as depression and bone loss, for example, and it makes sense to discuss all the possible options with your doctor before making the final decision.

Hormone replacement therapy

There are so many myths and half-truths relating to HRT, it is important to understand what it can and cannot do. It certainly cannot reverse or halt the ageing process or make a woman look years younger than her real age. However, if it eliminates problems such as hot flushes and broken nights, it can restore a woman's natural energy and vitality so that she feels as if she has shed a few years. Unlike the combined oral contraceptive (the pill), HRT medication does not usually contain synthetic hormones; it is mostly made from natural hormones derived from animal sources and contains smaller quantities of hormones than the pill that are designed to reproduce a woman's pre-menopausal hormonal levels. This means it can be taken safely by women for whom the pill was not suitable, either because it caused side effects or because they were already at an increased risk of thrombosis.

There are many forms of HRT, including skin patches, pills, creams and pessaries in varying combinations and doses of hormones, so if one type should prove unsuitable another might be more satisfactory. It may be necessary to go through a period of trial and error with different types of treatment to find the one that suits the individual woman best. A few women will not be able to use HRT for medical reasons and others prefer to avoid hormonal treatment altogether. In any case, if your symptoms are relatively minor or can be managed by other means, you may feel that you do not need it at all.

Many women are put off the whole idea of HRT because of scare stories in the media about associated health risks, but although possible risks do need to be considered carefully, many have been wildly exaggerated. These are summarized fully on page 65. When weighing up whether or not you want to begin HRT, you should obviously consider the possible benefits, both short- and long-term, as well as potential disadvantages for you personally, and your doctor or the staff at a menopause clinic should be able to provide you with all the information you need and give realistic advice. It is important that you are confident that taking HRT is the right course for you, otherwise you are less likely to stick with it once you have begun.

What is HRT?

As is clear from its name, the medication is designed to provide a substitute for those hormones that a woman's body produces in much reduced quantities from the menopause onwards. Prior to the cessation of her periods, as we have seen, levels will have been tailing off for some time, and they drop dramatically after the menopause, although small quantities of oestrogen are still secreted by fat cells and the adrenal glands. When HRT was first introduced in the last century, only oestrogen was given, until it was recognized that this treatment increased the risk of a woman developing cancer of the endometrium (the lining of the uterus). This problem was solved by adding progestogen (a synthetic form of progesterone) to protect the endometrium and this form of HRT is now prescribed for all women except those who have had their uterus surgically removed by a hysterectomy operation. Treatment may be prescribed on a short- or long-term basis, depending on circumstances and the woman's personal preference.

Different types of HRT

In its earliest days, back in the 1930s, oestrogen was given first by injection and then by pellets but neither of these methods of administration is used today. All HRT is oestrogen-based because it is the lack of this hormone that is responsible for menopause-related symptoms; the treatment is given because post-menopausal women are regarded as being in an oestrogen-deficient state.

Most women take oestrogen in combination with progestogen to induce a regular bleed in which the uterine lining is shed as in a normal menstrual period. Although most oestrogens used in HRT are natural, synthetic rather than natural progesterone is used because in its natural form its effects are short-lived and unreliable. It is added to the oestrogen component either as tablets or in patches combined with oestrogen. Depending on the particular regime prescribed, progestogen may be taken for part or all of each treatment cycle (see pages 59–60).

The hormones may be taken in a variety of forms and combinations, depending on the specific treatment being prescribed:

Oestrogen	Progestogen
Tablets	Tablets
Patches	Patches (together with oestrogen)
Implants	
Gels	
Creams	
Pessaries	
Vaginal rings	

There are various different ways of taking HRT and these different methods result in different bleeding patterns.

Cyclical or sequential therapy

This is the most widely prescribed 'regimen', as doctors call it, in which you take oestrogen every day and progestogen for part of each treatment cycle. The oestrogen may be given through a daily pill, a patch (which needs changing once or twice a week, depending on which one you're using), a gel applied daily to the skin or sometimes in the form of an implant. The progestogen can be taken in a pill or through a skin patch worn for 12–14 days. Over 90 per cent of women will have a regular monthly bleed shortly after the end of the progestogen treatment. There are also formulations that reduce the withdrawal bleeds to once every three months. Spotting may occur when you first begin treatment, but if you continue to bleed at other times the progestogen dose may need adjusting. You will probably be recommended this type of HRT if you begin therapy while peri-menopausal or within a year of your last period.

Many women prefer to use patches, which allow the hormones to be absorbed through the skin, so they do not have to worry about forgetting to take tablets. Some patches available now incorporate both oestrogen and progestogen; alternatively, you can opt for one consisting only of oestrogen which must be supplemented with progestogen tablets for a few days each month, unless you have had a hysterectomy. The latest types, called matrix patches, give better absorption and are smaller and thinner and almost invisible. They are also less likely to cause skin irritation than the traditional type of patch (called reservoir patches) because they do not contain alcohol.

Continuous combined therapy

Once you have not had a period for a year you can change to (or start on) this type of treatment, which eliminates the nuisance of bleeding for most women. It comes either as a skin patch or as tablets containing both oestrogen and progestogen which you take every day. You may experience some spotting or bleeding in the first few months, but the majority of women will eventually be free of withdrawal bleeds altogether. You may experience PMS symptoms, including breast tenderness, early on, but if they continue it is worth asking to try an alternative treatment which contains a different progestogen and so may suit you better.

Unopposed oestrogen

If you have had a hysterectomy, you can safely take oestrogen on its own in patch, tablet or gel formulations or as implants.

Local treatment

Women whose main problem during and after the menopause is vaginal dryness may prefer a local treatment such as oestrogen pessaries or creams absorbed through the vagina. There is also a device that works in a similar way: it consists of a ring which is inserted high in the vagina, where it releases small amounts of oestrogen for three months, after which it needs replacing.

Non-hormonal therapy

If you are anxious to avoid withdrawal bleeds, you might want to opt for an alternative to HRT which has many of the same health benefits. A treatment containing a synthetic compound called tibolone rather than oestrogen and progestogen is effective against menopausal symptoms and also provides some protection against osteoporosis.

Who needs HRT?

If your menopause arrives early – in your thirties or early forties – your doctor is likely to recommend that you start on HRT. This is because you would otherwise be exposed to the increased risk of osteoporosis and heart disease for a longer period than a woman who continues to produce oestrogen until she is around 50 years old. An early menopause can happen naturally to a minority of women, but it will also be inevitable once a woman has had her ovaries surgically removed. Having a hysterectomy is also likely to bring your menopause forward by around five years.

If your menopause begins around the average age, the severity of your symptoms will help you to determine whether and when it is right for you to take HRT, if this is what you want and your doctor agrees it would be appropriate. If your symptoms are mild or you feel you would prefer to cope

WHICH HRT METHOD IS BEST FOR YOU?

Method	Pros
Tablets	They are effective for emotional and physical symptoms, protect against osteoporosis and can be stopped straight away if you suffer side effects. Pills containing oestrogen, progestogen and testosterone are available.
Transdermal: patches and gels	They are effectively absorbed, offer good protection against osteoporosis, are easy to wear and simple to change. There are fewer side effects than with tablets because the hormone dose is lower. They can supply both oestrogen and progestogen, so oral progestogen does not have to be taken. Gels are easy to use and rarely cause skin irritation or side effects.
Subcutaneous HRT: implants	Effective control of both physical and emotional symptoms and very good protection against osteoporosis because the dosage is relatively high. Can be forgotten about for three to six months.
Local treatment: creams, pessaries and vaginal rings	Oestrogen in these forms is helpful both with vaginal dryness and irritation and with incontinence problems. They are easy to apply and can be used on their own for women who have few other symptoms or with other types of HRT if necessary.
Tibolone: tablets	Effective against menopausal symptoms and useful for those who cannot or prefer not to take hormones. It does not trigger withdrawal bleeds because the endometrium is not stimulated. Offers some protection against osteoporosis.

Cons

You have to remember to take them every day and, if you forget, you may experience spotting. Relatively large doses of hormones are needed because the pills are processed through the gut and liver, reducing the amount of hormone available for effective action. Nausea is more common than with other methods of administration and some women experience poor absorption, so the treatment is not sufficiently effective.

Some types may cause skin irritation in sensitive women, especially in hot weather. If your skin is dry or oily the patch can come off. Patches deliver a fixed dose of hormone, making adjustment more difficult. Gels need to be left for a few minutes to dry on the skin.

Difficult to alter the dosage if side effects occur and may be difficult to remove. Some women seem to develop a tolerance to the hormones so that symptoms recur even though hormone levels are high.

Creams and pessaries can be messy to apply, and the vaginal ring needs replacing after three months. If used for longer than a few weeks, local oestrogens will need to be supplemented with progestogen as some of the hormone will be absorbed into the bloodstream.

Some women experience spotting or bleeding; may not offer such effective protection against cardiovascular disease as oestrogen therapy. Only safe for women whose last period occurred 12 months before beginning treatment.

without medication, then self-help methods may be sufficient to improve your health and sense of wellbeing. If you are unsure, your doctor should be able to provide relevant information and advice to help you decide whether you want to try HRT.

There are two main reasons why you might want to opt for HRT: for the relief of troublesome symptoms and to protect yourself against the risk of osteoporosis and cardiovascular disease, which increases in the years following the menopause. HRT offers effective relief, often within a very short time of beginning treatment, against debilitating symptoms such as hot flushes and night sweats, vaginal dryness and painful intercourse, bladder problems, irritability and depression. You may also find that your memory, your ability to concentrate and make decisions, and your hair and skin recover some of their former 'life'. If you are in a relatively high-risk category for heart and blood-vessel disease or osteoporosis, you should consider the advantages of HRT very seriously even if you are not bothered much by menopausal symptoms.

Starting on HRT

You may be fortunate and find that HRT relieves your symptoms effectively with few side effects right from the word go. However, the majority of women who start taking it give up within a relatively short time – at present only 30 to 40 per cent of those who start taking HRT are still doing so a year later. Many dislike the idea of continuing to have 'periods', while others are put off by side effects. The secrets of success are to be as well informed as possible about what to expect and to find the combination of oestrogen and progestogen that suits you.

Achieving the correct balance can require an investment of time and patience by both you and your doctor to achieve the best results.

Side effects

When considering the (somewhat daunting) list of possible side effects, bear in mind that you may develop few or none of them, and it is often possible to alleviate them by adjusting your treatment:

- ❑ Nausea
- ❑ Headaches
- ❑ Irregular bleeding
- ❑ Premenstrual tension
- ❑ Depression
- ❑ Mood swings
- ❑ Tender or painful breasts
- ❑ Bloating/fluid retention
- ❑ Weight gain
- ❑ Abdominal cramps
- ❑ Greasy skin
- ❑ Aggressiveness
- ❑ Acne
- ❑ Tearfulness
- ❑ Loss of libido

If any of these symptoms are troublesome or persistent, always go back to your doctor, as it is likely that your treatment can be adjusted to reduce or eliminate them. Some, such as intermittent spotting or bleeding, usually ease with time, but otherwise changing the type or dose of progestogen may help.

If depression is related to HRT – which it may well not be – a switch from synthetic to natural progesterone may be the solution; new formulations are available which do not have to be taken by mouth, such as vaginal gels and suppositories. Similarly, you may find that headaches triggered by either the oestrogen or the progestogen component of HRT can be dealt with by lowering the dosage of either or switching to a different oestrogen or to natural progesterone. PMS is associated with the progestogen phase of combined therapy and switching to natural progesterone may help.

Doctors – and women – disagree about whether HRT is directly responsible for weight gain. It is difficult to be precise, because most women gain weight around the time of the menopause and afterwards anyway, and stored fat tends to be redistributed around the waist at this time.

The cancer risk

Despite frequent scare stories in the media, there is little evidence that taking HRT is associated with any increased risk of cancer. Since adding progestogen eliminated the increased risk of endometrial cancer associated with unopposed oestrogen, the main concern has been with breast cancer. Current medical opinion is that there is no increase in risk for the majority of women who take HRT for up to five years, although the risk may increase slightly beyond that. Women who are known to be at high risk because of a family history or other factors may choose not to take HRT, although many doctors now believe this is safe provided the women are carefully monitored. The potential risks and benefits must be weighed carefully by the individual woman and her doctor before a final decision is taken. Although there is no evidence that HRT plays a causative role in either ovarian or cervical cancer, the same cautious approach will be adopted by doctors when advising a woman who has previously had either of these conditions about whether HRT is safe for her.

Special concerns

Women with certain particular health problems should discuss the relative risks and benefits of taking HRT carefully with their doctor before going ahead. Severe liver disease may mean it is better to avoid oral treatment and opt instead for systems such as patches because that way the hormones do not pass through the liver. A doctor will also want to investigate any unusual vaginal bleeding before prescribing HRT. A possible cause is fibroids, which grow in the presence of oestrogen and need to be treated before hormone therapy is started. Other conditions, such as endometriosis and gallstones, may be aggravated by oestrogen, so HRT may not be the most appropriate treatment in these cases.

Continuing with HRT

As a general rule, doctors try not to prescribe medicine for longer than it is needed. This may be only days, as with antibiotics, or forever, as with insulin treatment for people with diabetes. The situation with HRT falls somewhere in between and the decision as to how long to remain on it involves weighing up the relative benefits and any possible risks on an individual basis. However, doctors generally recommend that you need to take HRT for a minimum of five years and possibly as many as ten to gain the best possible protection against osteoporosis and heart disease. Most women will find that the worst of their menopausal symptoms have subsided after two or three years on HRT, although some may need to continue treatment for up to five years. The decision to stop treatment should be taken in conjunction with your doctor, who will be able to advise you on the best way to tail off gradually.

Other orthodox treatment

If you cannot or do not wish to take hormone replacement therapy, there is a range of other medications available which can deal with some of the symptoms of the menopause. These are listed below.

Depression

Anti-depressant medication can usually alleviate the worst symptoms and lift your mood sufficiently for you to be able to consider 'talking' therapies to find the root of the problem if necessary. It is important to remember that while depression may be related to the hormonal changes which occur around the menopause, it can also develop for other reasons. Modern anti-depressants have few, usually minor, short-lived side effects and are not addictive, so don't hesitate to consult your doctor if you think you may be suffering from depression.

Anxiety

Tranquillizers are rarely prescribed these days because of the known risk of dependence, though sometimes a doctor may give a short course of medication to help someone through a particular crisis.

Insomnia

Sedative medication can help you get a good night's sleep, but it is not wise to become reliant on any kind of medication to deal with insomnia; it is much better, and healthier, to use natural methods (see page 75).

Hot flushes

Clonidine is a non-hormonal medication originally designed to treat raised blood pressure. It can reduce the frequency and severity of hot flushes, although it does not work for everyone. You may find it makes you drowsy, but it will have no effect on other hormone-related menopausal symptoms. Be sure to follow your doctor's advice when you stop taking it as you will need to tail off gradually to avoid any sudden rise in blood pressure. Your doctor may also suggest a drug called propranolol, which is normally used to treat high blood pressure, to relieve hot flushes.

PMS

Some women say that supplements of vitamin B6 (pyridoxine) help to relieve symptoms, although it is important not to take too much. A daily dose of 25–50mg is considered to be safe and you may need it only during the last two weeks of the cycle (two weeks before a period). Side effects can develop with higher doses taken over long periods, including skin sensitivity and rashes and nerve damage.

Gamma linolenic acid (GLA) may help to ease symptoms for some women. GLA is a breakdown product of cis-linolenic acid, an essential vegetable fatty acid found in sunflower, safflower and corn oils. It is difficult to determine dosage as each individual woman must find the level that suits her, but on average 500mg taken one to three times a day before menstruation is thought appropriate.

Osteoporosis

Vitamin D is necessary to keep bones and joints healthy and strong, and it encourages the absorption of phosphorus and calcium. It is manufactured in the body in response to sunlight on the skin and is also found in many foods (see page 108). Most women will get enough without needing to take supplements, unless their diet is poor or they are housebound. It cannot affect existing osteoporosis but a good intake is a useful preventive measure. There are a number of drug treatments available to promote bone density and treat osteoporosis which your doctor can prescribe if he or she thinks you could benefit from them.

Vaginal dryness

There are several brands of lubricant jelly that can be applied directly to the vagina to relieve this problem and make sexual intercourse more comfortable.

5 Complementary therapies

The growth in the popularity of complementary therapies over recent years has been phenomenal and the huge range of options can be confusing. Some, such as acupuncture and herbal medicine, have been used for centuries, while others, such as homoeopathy and Bach flower remedies, are of more recent origin. Many people turn to complementary therapies for help with chronic conditions that cannot be cured by orthodox medicine, while others use them to relieve stress or simply to enhance their overall sense of wellbeing.

One of the main attractions of complementary medicine is that it takes a holistic approach; in other words, its practitioners aim to treat the whole person and not just the symptoms or the disease itself. Side effects are rare and generally minor, although more caution will be needed with powerful therapies such as herbal medicine. Before you consult a complementary therapist, it is wise to discuss your plans with your doctor in case the complementary therapy would not be appropriate or would conflict with the conventional treatment that has already being prescribed. However, in most cases your doctor is likely to give the go-ahead – conventionally trained doctors are becoming much more open-minded about complementary therapies, even though some still adopt a sceptical approach.

Using complementary therapies

Generally, it is quite safe to use both complementary and conventional medicine at the same time. You should be wary of a complementary therapist who advises or encourages you to give up any existing conventional treatment and should not follow this advice without first consulting your doctor. Most therapists, however, will be happy to treat you in partnership with your doctor and will discuss any treatment you are currently receiving before treating you themselves. Many complementary therapies are suitable for self-treatment, but if at all possible it is best to consult a properly qualified practitioner, at least initially, to discuss how to go about treating yourself.

Around the time of the menopause, many women find themselves having to deal with issues such as fear of ageing and life changes such as children leaving home or relationship difficulties at the same time as suffering troublesome physical symptoms. Many find that complementary therapy enables them to cope better with both emotional and physical problems and helps them to remain calm and to feel in control when life is difficult. Restoring natural balance is a big theme of many types of complementary therapies and this makes them especially appropriate around the time of the menopause, when hormonal imbalances are a major source of trouble. Different therapists will approach the task of rebalancing in different ways, but all will focus on the individual woman and her personal, unique needs when devising a treatment plan.

Choosing a therapy

If you have never tried complementary therapy before, your best approach is to find out as much as you can about what's available and then simply start with the one that holds most appeal for you. You might want to consider whether you would prefer something relatively straightforward and practical, such as massage or osteopathy; or a more gentle treatment, such as aromatherapy or reflexology; or something with a more philosophical basis, such as yoga or acupuncture. Some people like the idea of remedies that can be seen as affecting the body directly, in which case homoeopathy, herbalism or Bach flower remedies would be a good choice.

If you are taking HRT or other medication you can continue to do so while having complementary treatment. Your therapist will ask you about current treatment, how you feel about it and whether it is effective. He or she will also want to know details of your general lifestyle, including your diet, work and sleep habits, emotional state and stress levels – in fact everything that might be contributing to your mental and physical health or lack of it. You should be prepared for a fairly lengthy question and answer session before any treatment begins since it is essential for the therapist to know as much as possible about you before deciding on the appropriate course of treatment.

Your choice of therapies may be limited depending on where you live; in some countries legislation controls what therapies are permitted. In general, however, there is no requirement for therapists to belong to a recognized professional body, although the majority probably do so voluntarily. This means it is up to you to check out the therapist of your choice: ask about what type of training they have had, how long it lasted and what qualifications they have. If they do belong to a professional organization, you may also want to contact them for advice. You can also contact such organizations to find a list of therapists in your area. When making contact with a practitioner, ask them to give an indication of what they charge for a treatment session and if you can have an initial consultation before you make a final decision about whether to have treatment.

When you meet the practitioner and have discussed your health and possible treatment, ask how many sessions you can expect to need, how frequent they should be and how soon you can expect to see results. Use the initial consultation to assess whether you feel this particular therapist is someone with whom you could establish a rapport and, most importantly, whether you have confidence and trust in him or her. While what you say about yourself and the details of your treatment are confidential, you may find that you share personal information with your therapist which you would not confide to even your nearest and dearest, so it is important that you feel completely comfortable about the idea of doing this before you begin. No responsible therapist will promise anything approaching a miracle cure, regardless of what your symptoms are, and you should distrust anyone who implies that this is a possibility.

Natural therapies

Aromatherapy

The word means 'treatment using scents' and refers to the use of essential oils derived from a variety of natural sources either individually or in combinations according to the needs of the person concerned. The oils are aromatic essences extracted from plants, flowers, trees, bark, grasses and seeds, each of which has its own distinctive therapeutic properties. They are often used in combination with carrier oils for massage, but may be added to bath water, inhalations, candles or skin sprays so that they are absorbed through the skin or inhaled, or both.

Many oils have more than one therapeutic quality: among the most beneficial are their antiseptic properties; their digestive and diuretic effects; their power to promote relaxation and pain relief; and their anti-inflammatory, anti-viral and anti-depression effects. Practitioners believe that the oils work both in a direct physical way and through their influence on the mind and the emotions. When the therapist has chosen or blended the oils appropriate for your needs, you will be asked whether the aroma appeals to you. Be honest – a scent that you dislike is unlikely to have the desired effect. It is important that you give the therapist full details of any condition, current treatment or allergies. This will influence the choice of oils, as some may not be suitable if you have certain conditions, such as raised blood pressure or epilepsy, for example. If you are opting to treat yourself, you should ideally consult a trained therapist first, but otherwise be sure to read the instructions, especially any warnings about conditions or medications that render a particular oil unsuitable for you. The other important cautionary note is that you must always check whether any essential oil you buy has already been diluted in carrier oil and, if it has not, do this yourself before applying it to your skin. You should never apply neat oil directly to your skin as it could cause an adverse reaction.

Essential oil of cypress is especially good for menopausal symptoms because it has cooling, drying qualities which help alleviate nervous tension, and a restful, woody smell. Use it in a burner or try adding it, together with a few drops each of clary sage, rosemary and lemon oils, to bath water. To make a cooling mist which will ease hot flushes, put 2 teaspoonfuls of cider vinegar into a spray bottle and top up with 100ml of still, bottled water, then add 3 drops each of cypress and clary sage essential oils, and shake before using.

Herbal medicine

There are two different schools of herbal medicine which, though based on similar principles, use different methods of diagnosis and different preparations: Western and Chinese herbalism. Both approaches, however, use the whole herb, in contrast to orthodox medicines, which frequently use extracts from plants or synthetic analogues. As with homoeopathy, herbal remedies are designed to support the body and promote its natural healing abilities. Herbal medicines come in a variety of forms, including tinctures, creams, compresses, tablets and capsules, or as infusions such as teas and decoctions. Chinese medicine has been used for over five thousand years and works on balancing the body's natural energy (called *chi*) and especially on equalizing the balance between the Yin and the Yang, which are often seen as female and male qualities.

The practitioner will choose remedies designed to work on specific imbalances to restore the person to wholeness in body, mind and spirit. You should not try to treat yourself but always consult a qualified practitioner, because the herbs can have powerful effects and wrongly used can be toxic. Usually you will be given selected herbs to prepare as drinks at home – and the taste can take some getting used to!

Popular treatments include *Nuo dao gen* and *Wu wei zi* for night sweats, *Quing huo* and *My dan pi* for hot flushes, *Bao shao yao* and *Sang shen zi* for hair loss and *Du fu zi* and *Chi shao yao* for dry, itchy skin.

Western herbalists also use plant remedies to restore balance and promote good health through enhancing what they call the 'vital force'. Stress, poor diet and pollution can weaken this force and illness is the result of its efforts to maintain harmony when the body is under threat. The aim of treatment is not merely to fight illness but also to prevent recurrences, detoxify the body and support the immune system.

St John's wort is a herbal remedy, which has long been used to treat depression, and which has been recently been shown in scientifically controlled studies to be extremely effective and to have few side effects. A popular medicine used by menopausal women is black cohosh, which is used to restore hormonal balance, thus helping to alleviate mood swings, depression, heavy bleeding and other symptoms related to oestrogen decline.

Homoeopathy

This therapy, devised in the nineteenth century by Dr Samuel Hahnemann, works on the principle that 'like cures like'. In other words, a substance that triggers certain symptoms when taken can also cure the same symptoms when they result from disease or illness. There are over two thousand different remedies, derived from vegetable, mineral and animal sources and prepared by a process of multiple dilutions and shakings. Finally the liquid, which retains no measurable trace of the original substance, is added to inert pills, which are then prescribed on an individual basis. The remedies are designed to stimulate and support the body's own healing systems, which means that symptoms may get worse before getting better. It's possible to treat yourself with homoeopathy, but a consultation with a qualified practitioner is likely to be more successful, as the remedies can then be tailored more specifically to your needs.

Lachesis, pulsatilla and amyl nit are among the most effective treatments for menopausal symptoms such as heavy bleeding, hot flushes and night sweats, and depression.

Acupuncture

Another element of traditional Chinese medicine, acupuncture is also based on the concept of restoring the free flow and balance of *chi*. This 'life force' is believed to flow along invisible channels in the body called meridians, and treatment is given by applying very fine needles to particular acupuncture points on the skin along the line of the meridians. Most people find the needles make the skin tingle but are not painful. It can be very helpful for symptoms such as migraine, hot flushes, heavy periods and poor skin tone, as well as for psychological problems such as poor memory and concentration.

Bach flower remedies

These are most appropriate for symptoms which are emotionally based. They were devised by Dr Bach with the aim of healing and eliminating the negative thoughts and feelings that can underlie both physical and mental symptoms. There are 38 different remedies, each tailored for a particular personality, attitude and state of mind, and they can be used individually or in combination. They can safely and effectively be used for home treatment and may enhance the benefits derived from other types of complementary therapy. Common menopausal remedies include walnut for life changes, mustard for unexplained depression, olive for fatigue, mimulus for fear of ageing, star of Bethlehem for sadness over lost youth and scleranthus for unexplained mood swings.

Chiropractic and osteopathy

These are both types of manipulative therapy and are similar, although slightly different techniques are used and chiropractors may concentrate more on the spine and nervous system. They can be very helpful for people with joint or muscle problems and poor skeletal alignment, and can also help to relieve tension, which results in emotional as well as physical symptoms. Like other complementary therapists, practitioners take a holistic approach and the techniques are generally neither violent nor painful. However, these therapies must be used with caution for anyone with osteoporosis and joint conditions such as arthritis.

Reflexology

A relatively modern form of treatment perfected during the last century, reflexology works by stimulating points on the feet or, sometimes, on the hands. Therapists visualize the feet and hands as a kind of mirror of the body, and every part of the body has its counterpoint on the feet and hands. The aim is to restore the proper balance of energy through the ten longitudinal zones which run from the extremities through the body to the head. By applying carefully placed pressure to the appropriate reflexes, therapists aim to improve overall physical and mental wellbeing, as well as to treat specific symptoms and conditions. Most people find the treatment sessions relaxing and enjoyable, and the practitioner may recommend simple methods of self-treatment to be used between sessions. Special attention is likely to be devoted to reflexes such as the pituitary, thyroid and adrenal glands in order to ease menopausal symptoms.

Massage

Traditional massage can not only relieve muscular tension, joint pains and general aches and discomfort but also work wonders in relieving stress and emotional problems. There are many different schools of massage which differ in both their techniques and their underlying philosophy. Your choice will depend on what holds the most appeal for you personally, as well as what is on offer in your area.

Traditional Swedish massage using oils on the skin is available almost everywhere and you may find other styles, such as Japanese shiatsu (or acupressure), Indian head massage or rolfing. Although you can learn simple techniques of self-massage, you really need to go to a qualified and experienced practitioner to gain the maximum benefits. Your therapist will need to know details of any existing health problems, such as arthritis or varicose veins, for example, as well as any menopausal symptoms, in order to treat you correctly. Mental and physical tension, headaches, bloating, period pains, mood swings, depression and irritability all respond well to massage and most people find that the whole experience is extremely relaxing and uplifting.

Hydrotherapy

As water is an important constituent in our body's make-up, it should not surprise us that it can be used therapeutically. It is vital to keep properly hydrated, which means drinking around 2.5 litres of water every day; this doesn't include tea and coffee, which actually deplete your system of water because they have diuretic properties. If you are losing a lot of fluid as a result of hot flushes and night sweats, keeping up your water intake is even more important. Among its many functions in the body, water helps to keep the skin moist and supple, lubricates the joints, keeps the digestive and elimination system working properly and maintains the natural cooling system.

As well as taking in water as a drink, you can use it in various forms of therapy to help boost your circulation and promote the elimination of toxins. Showering or sitting in alternate hot and cold water is food for the circulation, although you should not use this technique if you have a heart condition. Even something as simple as a hot-water bottle or an ice pack can be used to ease pain such as abdominal cramps and headaches.

Nutritional therapy

A nutritional therapist uses carefully selected diets to help promote optimum health, as well as to alleviate particular symptoms and conditions. You may believe that you already eat well, but a nutritional therapist will want to consider all aspects of your diet and lifestyle, together with any particular menopausal symptoms, before recommending changes to bring about health benefits. Despite the wide range of food available, many people in Western countries are overfed and undernourished at the same time, because they eat the wrong foods or have poor-quality diets. Some practitioners may use a range of techniques that they claim will diagnose allergies and food intolerance, sensitivity or deficiencies, but in general these are unreliable. Many allergies can be diagnosed by skin-patch or blood tests, but other methods are largely ineffective and usually inaccurate.

6 The food link

By choosing the right foods you can boost your overall health and sense of wellbeing and alleviate some of the symptoms of the menopause. Throughout life, a healthy, well-balanced diet is essential to maintain optimum functioning of all the systems in the body. As well as ensuring that you eat a varied range of foods, you should opt for natural foods whenever you can and keep processed food to a minimum. If your diet is balanced, it will provide you with all the vitamins and minerals you need.

Paying attention to your diet – being aware of what you are eating and how your body responds to food – is of the utmost importance. By adopting a healthy eating plan you will help maintain your weight at the right level for your height; this is important around the time of the menopause when women have a tendency to gain weight because of hormonal changes.

In the following pages, you will find the guidelines you need to ensure that your diet is as healthy as possible, but even if you already follow most of them, you will find suggestions as to some specific foods which have particular benefits as far as menopausal symptoms are concerned. If these are not already on your regular shopping list, it is worth adding them as they can play an important role in the production of natural oestrogen and help to regulate the hormonal fluctuations that occur at this time of bodily changes. You may find that they help to limit symptoms such as hot flushes, as well as improving your general physical and mental wellbeing during and after your menopause.

Changing your diet

When thinking about any changes you plan to make in your eating habits, bear in mind that your aim is to improve your hormone balance and avoid anything that will increase the effects of changing levels on the way you feel. Three important factors to consider are:

1 the amounts and types of fats and fibre in your diet;

2 foods which can contribute directly to levels of oestrogen and progesterone in your body;

3 the benefits of specific nutrients.

Our increased reliance on convenience and refined foods these days, together with the techniques of modern farming, have changed the quality of the food that most of us eat. Nutrients such as vitamins and minerals may be lost, wholly or partly, during refining and processing, and it is very easy to consume large amounts of substances which not only have no nutritional benefits but may even be counterproductive from a health point of view. For example, coffee, tea, cola drinks and alcohol all interfere with nutritional balance and may prevent you from obtaining all the essential nutrients your body needs to function properly. It goes without saying, of course, that smoking exacerbates the effects of a poor or unbalanced diet and again can prevent the proper absorption of vital nutrients such as vitamin C.

Drinking too much tea and coffee, eating too many sugary foods and snacks or having too many drinks that are high in sugar can result in fluctuating blood sugar levels, food cravings, headaches and fatigue. Cutting them back or changing to alternatives such as green tea, herbal teas, diluted fruit juice, fruit and yogurts will give you more energy and make you feel better.

Making a plan

It is all too easy to become so confused about what you are going to eat that you give up all attempts to change your diet before you have started. The best way to proceed is to draw up a menu plan, which you can then use to make shopping lists. You could start by devising an overall programme of the changes you plan to make during the next three months and base your detailed eating plan on this. At the end of the three months, if you have followed it fairly closely, you should begin to notice changes in the way you feel. Any menopausal symptoms are likely to improve over this period and this will encourage you to stick with your new way of eating.

Think of your three-month programme as a guide to getting the best from the food that you eat, without too many dramatic changes to begin with. Simply developing an awareness of which foods are good for you and which should be reduced or avoided is a big step in the right direction. Use the list below as a kind of route map and this will make it much easier for you to work your way through the detailed recommendations that follow.

Basic principles

❑ Drink six to eight glasses of water a day, preferably bottled or filtered.

❑ Eat at least five servings of fresh fruit and vegetables daily, raw or lightly cooked and organic if possible, to boost your vitamin and mineral intake.

❑ Reduce your intake of refined foods – sweets, cakes, biscuits, sugar, junk food, jam, puddings, chocolate and sugary drinks. Many people think of honey as being a naturally healthy food but although it may contain tiny quantities of minerals, it is really just another form of sugar with little in the way of nutrients.

❑ Choose low-fat dairy products and remember that you can also boost your calcium intake by eating more sardines, broccoli, salmon, lentils and nuts.

❑ Reduce your overall fat intake. Calories from fat should comprise no more than a third of your overall daily consumption. Be especially wary of 'hidden' fat in foods such as ready-made meals, crisps, pies and sausages and cut down on ordinary margarine and oils. Any fat which is solid at room temperature – for example, lard – is likely to be saturated fat; the same holds true for fat from animal sources, which includes butter and also the visible fat on meat. Choose lean meat or remove all fat before cooking.

Limit red meat to one or two portions a week. Try fish, poultry, pulses, nuts and rice (preferably brown) instead.

❏ The body does need some fat but the best types are polyunsaturated (oils such as corn oil, safflower, sunflower and soya bean oil) and monounsaturated (olive oil). Virgin cold-pressed olive oil tastes good and is ideal for cooking and salad dressings.

❏ Change to herb teas, green tea and dandelion coffee and cut back on ordinary tea and coffee, which contain the stimulant caffeine.

❏ Alcohol does you no harm in moderation and there is some evidence that a daily glass of wine may actually be good for you, but it is important not to overdo your consumption. Limit yourself to 3 units per day.

❏ Limit your salt intake and be aware of 'hidden' salt in foods such as packet soup, cereals and pickles.

Optimum nutrition

Many nutritionists and dieticians, as well as food scientists, now talk of 'nutriceuticals', which can be translated as meaning foods that have positive therapeutic and medicinal effects. The familiar expression 'you are what you eat' is true in the general sense that your health and wellbeing depend to a very great extent on what you put into your body.

While modern intensive farming methods and the availability of foods from all parts of the world, regardless of the season, have given us more choice than in any previous era, the production methods used, including hormones, fertilizers and pesticides, and the gap between harvesting or producing the food and its consumption may reduce its nutritional value. Nevertheless, by taking care when planning menus, you can ensure your meals are healthy and well balanced, as well as being enjoyable.

To make healthy eating easier, it is useful to take account of the various food 'groups' which need to be included in your diet. These are carbohydrates, proteins, fruit and vegetables, fats, vitamins and minerals, and together they comprise the basic components of a nutritious and balanced diet.

Carbohydrates

Most nutritionists agree that carbohydrates should provide around 60 per cent of daily calories, but the picture is slightly complicated by the fact that they come in two forms. The more desirable are complex carbohydrates, such as root vegetables, cereals, rice, pulses and legumes, pasta and some fruits. It is better to opt for the unrefined forms – wholemeal bread, rice, pasta and breakfast cereals, for example – because much of the nutritional content is lost when these foods are refined into their 'white' form. The unrefined versions are also broken down more slowly in the gut, which means they release energy (glucose) into the bloodstream at a slow rate. This is not the case with simple carbohydrates, such as sugar, which produce a rapid rise in blood glucose levels, stimulating the release of insulin from the pancreas, which causes blood glucose to fall with equal rapidity.

Proteins

These are often called the body's building blocks, but you need fewer of them than you might think. They should provide no more than 15 per cent of your daily calorie consumption. All the main organs of the body are created from protein; skin, bone, muscle tissue and hair all contain protein and they are important for the effective functioning of the immune system. When you eat large amounts of protein, the body stores the excess in muscles and organs. Protein is broken down into amino acids by enzymes during digestion and these are absorbed into the bloodstream and used to repair tissue and muscles. Good sources include meat, fish, poultry, nuts, dairy produce and pulses.

Fruit and vegetables

These are absolutely vital to maintain good health and contain many natural chemicals which help to protect against a wide range of illnesses. You should eat at least five portions a day (remember potatoes do not count as vegetables) to ensure that you meet your body's vitamin requirements; the more fresh fruit and vegetables you consume, the less likely it is that you will need to take vitamin supplements in addition to your diet. Of particular importance are the antioxidant vitamins and minerals, vitamins C, E, beta-carotene (which is converted into vitamin A in the body) and selenium, a trace mineral found in the soil. These are known to promote good health and protect from disease by aiding the body's natural defences against damage by free radicals – chemicals produced naturally in the body which limit the effectiveness of the immune system. The so-called 'ACE' vitamins are provided by making sure that you include in your diet dark, leafy vegetables such as broccoli and spinach and yellow-orange fruits and vegetables such as apricots, mangoes, carrots, sweet potatoes, red peppers, citrus fruits and avocados.

ANTIOXIDANTS

Antioxidants (vitamins C, E and beta-carotene, a precursor of vitamin A) help to control the unstable molecules called free radicals that, when produced in excess, can attack and damage various cells in the body. Sunlight, smoking, illness, pollution and stress can trigger over-production of free radicals. As well as damaging the cellular structure of arteries and other tissue, they may affect collagen so that skin starts to look leathery and tough, creating wrinkles, creases and bags under the eyes. Antioxidants are believed to slow down the damage caused by free radicals and are present in minerals such as selenium, zinc, manganese and iron, as well as in the 'ACE' vitamins. Green tea is a good source of antioxidants and is a refreshing drink, especially if you are trying to cut down on your consumption of ordinary tea and coffee.

All fruit and vegetables should be thoroughly washed before cooking or eating raw to remove any chemicals on the skin, although if you opt for organically grown produce this should not be a problem.

Fibre

Fibre is a natural component of all plant-derived foods and comes from the cell walls. Although it has no nutritional value, it is essential for efficient digestion and elimination of waste products. It is important because it absorbs water from the digestive tract, making stools bulkier so they pass out through the body more smoothly and comfortably. Increasing the amount of fibre in your diet will also mean that glucose from the food you have eaten will be released into your bloodstream gradually rather than in a rush. There are two types of fibre: soluble – from fruit, vegetables, pulse, and oats, for example; and insoluble – unrefined rice, nuts, fruit peel and bran. Some foods contain both types. Another advantage for those trying to control their weight is that a high-fibre diet helps you to feel full. In the past, bran was promoted as a good source of fibre, but because it is a refined food it can interfere with the effective absorption of nutrients such as zinc, magnesium and calcium. For this reason it is better to get your fibre from wholegrains, fruit, pulses and legumes, and vegetables. If your diet has previously been low in fibre, you should increase the amount you eat gradually to avoid 'wind' and indigestion, and make sure you drink plenty of water. Good sources of fibre include:

- ❏ cooked and raw fresh fruit and vegetables;
- ❏ wholegrains such as brown rice, wholegrain crackers, wholemeal bread, wholemeal pasta, beans, nuts and seeds;
- ❏ muesli – try soaking it overnight to make it easier for your system to absorb the necessary nutrients.

Fats

Fats are an essential part of a healthy diet but you need to know which ones are beneficial to health and which ones are not. Most foods contain varying amounts of saturated, polyunsaturated and monounsaturated fats.

Saturated fats derived mainly from animal sources, these are found in such foods as meat, butter, full-fat milk, lard and cheese, as well as coconut oil, margarine and processed meat products such as sausages, salami, burgers, pâté and bacon. They contribute to obesity due to their high calorie content and can also increase blood cholesterol levels and encourage the development of atheroma, which can clog up arteries.

Trans-fatty acids these fats are found in many hard margarines and spreads, as well as in processed foods such as pies, crisps, biscuits, cakes and some meat and dairy products. There have been suggestions that trans-fatty acids might be harmful because they trigger the production of free radicals – molecules that can damage cell structure. They are also linked to other health problems such as obesity, furring of the arteries and high levels of cholesterol.

Polyunsaturated fats these are found in oily fish, nuts, seeds and some vegetables. There are two basic types, omega-6 (linoleic acid) and omega-3 (linolenic acid), both of which perform several essential roles within the body. Omega-6 EFAs (essential fatty acids) are found in nuts, seeds and vegetable oils, especially corn, safflower, soya, sunflower and walnut oils. Omega-3 EFAs are present in oily fish, such as mackerel, herrings and sardines, and in walnuts and rapeseed oil. These oils are particularly important in keeping skin from becoming dry and they help to maintain a healthy metabolism and good joint mobility. They contribute to preventing heart disease – an increased risk for post-menopausal women – by reducing the blood's tendency to clot. They also play a vital part in maintaining a healthy nervous system and immune system and promote good fluid balance in the body, which may help with symptoms such as fluid retention. Linseed (flax) oil is a particularly rich source of EFAs and contains beta-carotene and vitamin E. It is not suitable for cooking but makes a delicious addition to salads and can also be mixed with other foods, especially yogurt.

Monounsaturated fats sometimes known as omega-9, are a useful substitute for saturated fats and some also contain EFAs. Olive oil is the best known, but other sources include avocados, nuts, seeds and rapeseed oil. The relatively low rates of cardiovascular disease in some Mediterranean countries have been ascribed in part to high consumption of olive oil, although it is likely that other factors are also relevant.

Oils

When choosing oils, opt for the very best quality you can afford, as they will be the purest and least processed and thus offer more potential health benefits. Extra virgin olive oil, which is generally unrefined, and cold-pressed organic unrefined oils are the best choices. Unrefined oil is extracted without the use of heat, unlike sunflower oil, for example, and heat affects the quality and nutritional content, thus lowering the potential health benefits. You need to think about where you keep your oil, because it can be attacked by free radicals which causes oxidation. Store, preferably in dark rather than clear bottles, away from heat and sunlight, and don't overheat it when cooking.

Fat sense

For all their bad reputation as promoters of weight gain, as we have seen, fats are an essential component of our diet. The secret to getting the right balance is to choose them carefully and then use them sparingly.

Do:

❏ Spread butter thinly or replace your usual brand with an unsaturated spread.

❏ Choose semi-skimmed or skimmed rather than full-fat milk.

❏ Trim off excess fat on meat and use leans cut whenever possible.

❏ Cook with liquid fats, preferably virgin olive oil, and use sparingly as salad dressings.

❏ Read food labels carefully – saturated fats are in many products, particularly refined and processed foods.

❏ Avoid or minimize your consumption of hidden saturated fats in cakes, biscuits and pastries.

❏ Grill rather than fry food.

❏ Regularly replace meat with fish, lentils and nuts.

Don't:

❏ Heat oils to too high a temperature.

❏ Roast nuts – it destroys the nutrients in the oils.

❏ Use hydrogenated margarine or those made with polyunsaturated vegetable oils that have been hydrogenated.

❏ Store oils in the light, for example in clear bottles on the windowsill.

Phytoestrogens

Phytoestrogens are plant foods that produce natural oestrogens and are similar in structure to the female hormone (the word *phyto* is Greek and means plant). They have about 1 per cent of the potency of our own oestrogen and can raise or lower oestrogen levels in the female body. In comparison with HRT they provide much less oestrogen, but they may nevertheless help to counteract the fall in levels that occurs at the time of the menopause. Phytoestrogens may also help to protect against heart disease and osteoporosis and are therefore important at this stage in a woman's life.

Most fruit, cereals and vegetables contain phytoestrogen in varying strengths. Those containing isoflavones are the most beneficial. These are found in legumes such as soya, chickpeas and lentils.

Until recently, it was believed that the high soya content of the Japanese diet was the reason why women in that country appeared to have fewer menopausal symptoms and less breast cancer than women who follow a Western diet. However, new research has questioned this assumption and it is now thought that the high fish intake in Japan might be the reason, though some soya consumption may still offer health benefits.

Sources of phytoestrogens and isoflavones

fruits apples, bananas, cherries, citrus fruits, cranberries, dates, figs, papaya, pomegranates, plums, rhubarb.
grains barley, oats, rice, rye, wheat.
herbs and spices fennel, parsley, red clover, sage and cinnamon.

pulses and legumes aduki beans, chickpeas, kidney beans, lentils, peas.

seaweed kelp, kombu, nori, wakame.

seeds caraway, linseed, pumpkin, poppy, sunflower.

soya and soya products miso (fermented soya beans used as flavouring for soups and casseroles), soya milk, tofu, soya flour.

sprouts alfalfa, mung beans.

vegetables beetroot, broccoli, carrots, celery, fennel, garlic, green beans, potatoes, yam.

The benefits of phytoestrogens

Research on the effects of soya has suggested that it may help to reduce hot flushes and night sweats, as well as reducing vaginal dryness and irritation. Soya beans have been found to contain at least five compounds believed to inhibit cancer, one of which is chemically similar to the drug tamoxifen, prescribed for women who have had oestrogen-dependent breast cancer to prevent a recurrence. The phytoestrogens and tamoxifen are believed to work in a similar way: that is, locking on to the oestrogen receptors and thus inhibiting cancer growth. Research is currently being undertaken to find out whether increasing the intake of phytoestrogens and isoflavones helps protect against breast cancer and osteoporosis. Some studies have indicated that soya may help to activate bone growth and therefore improve bone density, but further work is needed to establish whether it can play a role in preventing osteoporosis.

Phytoestrogens are also linked to the reduction of cholesterol in the body. Cholesterol is a blood fat that is found in all body tissues and is a constituent of atheroma, the fatty substance that can clog up arteries. The amount of cholesterol in your blood depends upon many factors, such as your age, diet, sex and lifestyle, but most importantly on your genetic inheritance. There are two main forms: high-density lipid (HDL) and low-density lipid (LDL). The former is carried in the bloodstream to the liver for breakdown, while the latter is taken to the organs and tissues for use. LDL is the type that may stick to artery walls and impede blood flow. Before the menopause women usually have higher levels of HDL in their bloodstream and low levels of LDL, but after the menopause the balance alters, increasing the risk of heart disease. Raising oestrogen levels can help reduce the risk significantly because it shifts the cholesterol balance in favour of HDL.

Although heredity is the most important factor in determining cholesterol levels, eating saturated fats can raise the level of LDL and foods containing phytoestrogens may help to lower them.

Stress-busting foods

The adrenal glands that sit above the kidneys have many functions. They manufacture 28 individual hormones, help with the digestion of food, regulate the thyroid gland, top up energy levels and help the body to deal with stress. They also produce small amounts of oestrogen, which becomes more important after the menopause when ovarian production stops. Stress causes the body to use up its resources of minerals and vitamins rapidly. When you are in a situation that triggers stress, the adrenals release adrenaline and noradrenaline – the so-called stress hormones – to prepare you for tackling the 'danger' by fight or flight. As the situation is resolved, the

SEAWEED

Sometimes known as sea vegetable, seaweed is very low in calories and has a high mineral content, containing zinc, chromium, selenium, manganese, magnesium, calcium, iron and iodine. The latter is very important in helping to maintain a healthy thyroid gland, which regulates the metabolism. As the metabolic rate slows after the menopause, seaweed can be a useful addition to your diet; use it to flavour stews and soups. Many varieties are available in health food shops, including:

○ agar – sold in flake form; very high in fibre;

○ hijiki – looks like tangled black string and tastes like liquorice; half a cup of cooked hijiki contains as much calcium as half a cup of milk;

○ kombu – kelp, with a sweet/salty taste; high in magnesium, potassium, calcium, iron and iodine; can be toasted for snacks or sprinkled on other dishes;

○ nori – sea lettuce, nutty-tasting and high in vitamins A and B; comes in sheets and you can wrap other food, such as rice, in it;

○ wakame – a dark green leaf, it is a rich source of vitamins A, B complex and E.

adrenals return to normal, but if it is not resolved, production of stress hormones continues. In the long term, raised levels of stress hormones may interfere with the effective function of the immune system and leave you feeling tired, weak and sometimes completely fatigued.

Stress seems to be an inevitable part of life for most people today, whether it's mental or physical, and poor nutrition exacerbates its effects. Eating well will help your adrenal glands to function properly and your body to cope with the strains placed upon it by stressful situations and lifestyles. A good intake of vitamins and minerals is particularly important around the menopause as the body adapts to the hormonal changes taking place. Prolonged stress may deplete your body of important minerals such as magnesium, zinc, calcium, sodium, potassium and copper. Keep up your levels by eating a mineral-rich diet, including dark green vegetables, yellow-orange vegetables and fruit, legumes, pulses, wholegrains, eggs and meat.

Sodium

The body needs sodium, but high levels of this mineral can be associated with raised blood pressure and affect the body's ability to balance fluid retention. Sodium chloride (common salt) is a major source of sodium in our bodies and the average Western diet contains large amounts; most people probably consume ten times more salt than they need. Many foods, such as fruit, vegetables and grains, already contain sodium, so adding salt to the diet to provide sodium is unnecessary.

Convenience and refined foods contain more salt than most people realize: burgers, biscuits, pizza, ketchup and salad dressings are just some of the culprits with high salt levels. By opting for fresh food instead, you can decrease your salt intake significantly. Avoid adding salt to the water when cooking vegetables, for example, and do not put extra on your food at the table. When you are shopping it is worth develop the habit of checking food labels for salt content.

Controlling weight and mood swings

Maintaining a healthy weight is important at any age but especially during and after the menopause, when there is a tendency to put on weight. Keeping active and taking regular exercise will help to maintain a weight that is right for you. Excess weight not only feels uncomfortable, but can lead to many healh complications and increases the risk of heart disease and diabetes.

However, a small increase in weight during the menopause is acceptable because it helps to prevent oestrogen levels from falling too far. As the ovaries stop production, so the body fat acts as a supplementary source of oestrogen. Eating a healthy

---

TIPS FOR HEALTHY WEIGHT LOSS

- ○ Eat plenty of fresh fruit and vegetables, which are high in vitamins and low in calories.
- ○ Increase fibre-rich foods such as fruit, vegetables, whole grains, beans and lentils.
- ○ Eat more fish, poultry and lean meat.
- ○ Avoid fried food.
- ○ Cut down on fatty meat products such as sausages, pork pies and sausage rolls.
- ○ Reserve cakes and pastries for special occasions.
- ○ Choose low-fat dairy options.
- ○ Drink plenty of water.
- ○ Try to cut back on stimulants such as coffee and tea.
- ○ Avoid alcoholic drinks – they are high in calories.
- ○ Enjoy your food.

---

diet will keep your weight within acceptable limits and you may even find you lose a little. The food we consume is converted into energy or fat, and by eating the right types of food we can encourage out bodies to use it rather than store it as fat.

The best types of food for energy are the complex carbohydrates, because as well as supplying energy they also keep blood sugars steady, which will help to prevent mood swings. To lose weight you have to consume less energy than you expend and changing your eating habits for good is always going to be preferable to going on crash diets. The latter can provide only a temporary solution, because after an initial loss you are virtually certain to put it back on again once you resume your old eating habits.

Food allergies and intolerance

Adverse reactions to certain foods seem to be increasingly common, but it is important to distinguish between the various types. If you are allergic to particular foods, your body will react to them as if they were an alien invader such as a bacterium or virus. The immune system produces antibodies to fight off the invasion and in extreme cases this can result in a potentially fatal reaction known as anaphylactic shock. More commonly, however, an allergy results in symptoms such as skin rashes or eruptions, nausea and vomiting, and diarrhoea. People who are intolerant to a particular food usually have a reaction because their body lacks the ability to digest it properly; the most common examples are lactose intolerance (inability to digest milk protein) and coeliac disease (inability to digest gluten, a protein in wheat). Such conditions arise because the person lacks the digestive enzyme needed to process something in the particular food and symptoms may include serious digestive problems.

Food sensitivity is much more common and though unpleasant is not life-threatening. Symptoms may be vague but can include bloating, water retention, aching joints, digestive and skin problems, asthma, hyperactivity and migraine headaches. Often it turns out that the problem food is one you tend to crave. Cutting out suspect foods for a period may help identify the culprit(s), though this can be a difficult and time-consuming process. Stop eating all the foods you think may be troubling you for about three weeks, then reintroduce them one by one to see which causes a reaction. When you first cut them out you may find that you feel worse as you suffer withdrawal symptoms. If you add a food and it produces the reaction, take it back out again and wait until you stabilize before reintroducing another food. A qualified nutritionist wil be able to advise you, and can help you to devise a suitable programme to follow.

Common culprit foods in allergies and intolerances

❑ Alcohol

❑ Chocolate

❑ Citrus fruits

❑ Coffee and caffeinated drinks such as chocolate, cocoa, cola and tea

❑ Dairy products

❑ Honey

❑ Peanuts

- ❏ Pickles and pickled products
- ❏ Processed and smoked meats, including bacon, frankfurters and salami
- ❏ Shellfish
- ❏ Smoked fish
- ❏ Spices and flavour enhancers such as monosodium glutamate (MSG)
- ❏ Strawberries
- ❏ Wheat and wheat products, including bread, cereals and pasta
- ❏ Yeast

Poor eating habits

Irregular meals, missing meals and low blood glucose levels can affect not only your health but also your moods. Eating little and often helps to stabilize blood glucose and it is important not to miss breakfast as blood glucose falls overnight. Complex carbohydrates are the ideal foods to keep blood glucose levels stable as they release energy slowly into the bloodstream. A banana or a slice of wholemeal toast is a good choice for a quick snack whenever you are feeling hungry.

Water is essential to maintain optimum health because it keeps the body properly hydrated; try to remember to drink water throughout the day, as by the time you start to feel thirsty you are already dehydrated. Water flushes toxins from the body, stopping it becoming sluggish, cleans the system and repairs the cells. It helps to keep skin looking and feeling good from the inside out. Filtered or bottled mineral water is best and certain varieties contain trace minerals that are important for maintaining health.

ESSENTIAL VITAMINS AND MINERALS

Nutrient	Food sources	Benefits
Vitamin A	Liver; eggs; carrots; spinach; broccoli; fruit	Eyesight; skin; possible protection against cancer
Vitamin C	Peppers; oranges; strawberries; blackcurrants	Helps heal wounds; may fight colds, flu and infections; protects gums; keeps joints and ligaments in good working order; antioxidant
Vitamin D	Tuna; salmon; mackerel; sardines; fish-liver oils; egg yolks	Aids absorption of calcium and phosphorus for healthy bones and teeth
Vitamin E	Green leafy vegetables; corn; avocado; asparagus; wheatgerm; wholegrain cereals; brown rice; pure vegetable oils; nuts; seeds; soya beans; tofu	Cell growth; antioxidant
Vitamin B1	Most foods including wheatgerm; wholegrain cereals; pulses; nuts	Helps the breakdown of carbohydrates; nervous system
Vitamin B2	Liver; kidney; dairy produce; eggs; brewer's yeast; wheat bran; wheatgerm	Repairs body tissue
Vitamin B3	Fish; wheatgerm; wholegrain cereals	Essential for chemical reactions
Vitamin B6	Lean meat; liver; fish; wholegrains; bananas; avocados; potatoes	Nervous system; skin; red blood cells
Vitamin B12	Liver; kidney; some fish; shellfish; eggs; milk	Blood and nerves

Nutrient	Food sources	Benefits
Vitamin K	Most vegetables, especially dark green leafy ones; liver	Helps in the production of some proteins
Calcium	Red meat; liver; oily fish; wholegrain cereals; leafy green vegetables	Bones, teeth and nails; muscles and nerve function
Copper	Turnips; peaches; shellfish; nuts; lentils	Helps prevent osteoporosis; antioxidant
Iron	Lean red meat; liver; pulses; dark green leafy vegetables; dried fruit	Makes haemoglobin, the pigment in red blood cells that helps transport oxygen around the body
Magnesium	Lean meat; fish; shellfish; pulses; brown rice; green vegetables; bananas; nuts; seeds	Regulates thyroid hormones and protects against artery clogging; cancels out the pollutants in the body
Potassium	Bananas; citrus fruits; dried fruits; nuts; seeds; potatoes; pulses	Keeps up energy levels – releases energy from the muscles; stops blood sugar fluctuations which can cause dizziness and tiredness; needed for production of cells, bone, proteins and fatty acids
Selenium	Lean meat; liver; fish; shellfish; brazil nuts; wholegrain cereals; tomatoes; broccoli; onions	Maintains normal blood pressure and regular heartbeat; facilitates transmission of nerve impulses
Zinc	Red meat; sardines; shellfish; root vegetables; nuts; seeds	Boosts immune system; improves red blood cells

NUTRIENTS ESSENTIAL FOR GOOD SKIN

Nutrient	What it does
Vitamin A	Antioxidant; helps to slow down the accumulation of keratin and keep the skin supple
Beta-carotene (pro-vitamin A)	Provides the body with the components to manufacture vitamin A; protects against the ageing effects of ultraviolet light and boosts immunity
Bioflavonoids	Antioxidant; slows down the deterioration of connective tissue and strengthens the small capillaries that feed the skin. Strengthens capillaries, preserves collagen, protects against osteoporosis, strengthens walls of vagina, promotes healthy cell structures
Vitamin B2	Necessary for the development and repair of healthy skin tissue
Vitamin B3	Helps the skin produce natural sunscreening substances, such as melanin
Vitamin B5 (panthothenic acid)	Necessary for the formation of new skin tissue to maintain healthy hair
Vitamin B6	Helps maintain normal oil balance in the skin and prevent allergic reactions; helps immune and nervous system
Vitamin B12	Helps the blood carry oxygen to the skin; helps eliminate toxins
Biotin	Helps the body use essential fats; moderates the output of overactive sebaceous glands
Vitamin C	Antioxidant, so helps protect against free radicals; helps manufacture collagen; anti-bacterial, so helps to reduce infection on the skin; detoxifies, helping to eliminate waste; vital for production of collagen

Where to find it	Protects against
Oily fish; offal; eggs; dairy foods; orange and yellow fruits, including peaches	Scaly skin; flaky scalp; acne; poor wound healing
Carrots; dark green vegetables; apricots; oranges; tomatoes; peppers; sweet potatoes; squash; pumpkin; watercress; cabbage; broccoli	As for vitamin A
Pith and segments of citrus fruits; apricots; blackberries; cherries; rose hips; apples; buckwheat	Easy bruising; slow wound healing; premature ageing
Milk; eggs; cereals; liver; green leafy vegetables; mackerel; mushrooms	Seborrhoeic dermatitis or inflammation around the nose and mouth; cracked lips; dull or oily hair
Brown rice; chicken; wheatgerm; tuna; broccoli	Dermatitis; acne; eczema; fatigue; depression
Yeast; liver; kidney; eggs; brown rice; wholegrain cereals; lentils; wholemeal bread; nuts; dried fruits	Muscle tremors; cramps; fatigue; anxiety
Chicken; yeast extract; broccoli; bananas; wheatgerm; beef; fish; eggs; brown rice; nuts; soya beans; whole grains	Overactive sebaceous glands, resulting in oily skin; flaky skin; water retention
Red meat; liver; eggs; fish	Dry skin; dermatitis; pale complexion
Offal; wheatgerm; brewer's yeast	Dry skin; eczema; scaly dermatitis
Most fruit and vegetables: blackcurrants; oranges; peppers; cherries; strawberries; broccoli; watercress	Broken thread veins; rough, scaly skin; easy bruising; red pimples; dry scalp

NUTRIENTS ESSENTIAL FOR GOOD SKIN cont.

Nutrient	What it does
Vitamin E (tocopherol)	Helps prevent cell damage; strengthens blood vessels; maintains good circulation; antioxidant which helps to protect against oxidation of polyunsaturated fat cells in cell membranes; especially important if diet is rich in fish and polyunsaturated fats
Folic acid	Slows down the loss of moisture from the skin
Calcium	Helps skin regeneration; maintains good acid-alkaline balance; helps prevent osteoporosis, essential for strong bones
Magnesium	Works with calcium to build and slow down the age-related shrinkage that produces wrinkles; essential for muscle activity; aids absorption of calcium to produce strong bones, needed to help prevent osteoporosis
Selenium	Antioxidant, so fights free radicals; helps body use vitamin E; reduces inflammation
Silica	Needed for collagen manufacture
Sulphur	Fights bacterial infection to help keep skin clear; aids detoxification by stimulating bile secretion
Co-enzyme Q10	Supports immune system, so fights bacterial infection; antioxidant, so slows ageing caused by free radicals
Zinc	Antioxidant; helps to make the protein that carries vitamin A to the skin; slows down the age-related weakening of collagen and elastin fibres; supports the immune system in destroying bacteria; helps strengthen bones

Where to find it	Protects against
Seeds; nuts; oily fish; sunflower oil; avocado; beans; wheatgerm	Premature wrinkles; pale skin; acne; easy bruising; slow wound healing
Brewer's yeast; liver; wheatgerm; molasses; green leafy vegetables; eggs; nuts; wholegrains	Dry skin; eczema; cracked lips; pale complexion
Milk; cheese; yogurt; almonds; parsley; brewer's yeast; sesame seeds; kale; seaweed; turnips; almonds; soya beans; dandelion leaves; hazelnuts; honey; horseradish; salmon; dairy products	Sallow, 'tired' skin
Fresh green vegetables; raw wheatgerm; soya beans; milk; wholegrains; seafood; figs; apples; oily fish; nuts	Constipation, producing sallow and blemished skin; bone shrinkage; lack of energy
Herrings; molasses; tuna; oysters; mushrooms; wheatgerm; bran; onions; broccoli; shellfish	Dull complexion; dry skin
Horsetail (herb)	Premature wrinkles; eczema; psoriasis; acne; poor wound healing
Lean beef; dried beans; fish; eggs; cabbage	Dull complexion; skin infections; fatigue
Soya oils; sardines; mackerel; peanuts; pork	Depressed immunity; sallow skin
Meat; wholegrains; brewer's yeast; wheatbran; wheatgerm; soy lecithin; beans; apricots; peaches; oysters; mustard seeds; cocoa; pumpkin seeds; nectarines; eggs	Dull complexion; eczema; acne; limp, dull hair; white marks on fingernails

Supplements

Making the time to shop and prepare meals from scratch is not always easy, which is why we sometimes resort to convenience foods and take-aways. The danger there is that poor eating habits can result in a deficiency in essential nutrients. A massive industry has grown up to provide supplements, but the choice on offer in supermarkets, pharmacies and health food shops is vast and often confusing.

If you suspect you should be taking supplements, it is worth asking your doctor to refer you to a qualified dietician for expert advice. In particular, you should be wary of any products that claim to treat or cure specific conditions or serious symptoms. Ideally, you should not need to take supplements if you are eating a healthy, balanced and varied diet, and nutrients absorbed in their natural form from good food are far more beneficial than synthetic substitutes.

7 Recipes

This chapter contains recipes that have been chosen to alleviate many of the symptoms experienced during the menopause. You may be surprised to learn that simple changes to your diet can make a difference. Many people are afraid that healthy eating will be time-consuming and will mean cutting out the foods that they enjoy. This certainly does not have to be the case, as the recipes included in this chapter use fresh produce that is readily available in any supermarket, they are simple to prepare and are delicious too. There are plenty of recipes to choose from including soups, stir-fries, salads, pasta and risottos.

Each recipe has been nutritionally analysed to include the calories and kilojoules, grams of protein, carbohydrate, saturated fat and fibre.

Soups and starters

Carrot and sage soup

alcohol free ✓ | citrus free ✓ | dairy free ✗ | gluten free ✓ | wheat free ✓

Serves 6
Preparation time: 15 minutes
Cooking time: about 1 hour

Per serving
Energy 87 kcals/363 kJ | Protein 1 g | Carbohydrate 12 g | Fat 4 g
Saturated fat 2 g | Fibre 4 g

25 g (1 oz) butter
1 large onion, finely chopped
750 g (1½ lb) carrots, thinly sliced
900 ml (1½ pints) vegetable stock
1 tablespoon chopped sage leaves
salt and pepper
sage sprigs, to garnish (optional)

1 Melt the butter in a large heavy pan, add the onion and fry
gently until soft but not golden, then add the carrots and stock.
Season with salt and pepper. Bring to the boil and simmer,
uncovered, for about 30 minutes.

2 Purée the soup in a food processor or blender until smooth, then
return to the rinsed pan and add the chopped sage. Bring to the
boil and simmer for another 15 minutes.

3 Serve the soup garnished with sage sprigs, if you like.

Carrot and coriander noodle soup

alcohol free ✓ | citrus free ✗ | dairy free ✓ | gluten free ✗ | wheat free ✗

Serves 4
Preparation time: 10 minutes
Cooking time: about 40 minutes

Per serving
Energy 163 kcals/682 kJ | Protein 3 g | Carbohydrate 29 g | Fat 5 g
Saturated fat 1 g | Fibre 6 g

1 tablespoon vegetable oil
1 onion, chopped
750 g (1½ lb) carrots, finely chopped
1 teaspoon ground coriander
150 ml (¼ pint) orange juice
1 litre (1¾ pints) hot vegetable stock
50 g (2 oz) dried egg thread noodles
3 tablespoons chopped coriander
salt and pepper

1 Heat the oil in a large saucepan and fry the onion for 3 minutes until softened. Add the carrots, stir in the coriander and fry for 5 minutes. Add the orange juice and 900 ml (1½ pints) of the stock and bring to the boil, then simmer for 30 minutes.

2 Meanwhile, bring a large saucepan of water to the boil. Add the noodles, stir well and then cover the pan. Remove from the heat and set aside for 6 minutes. Drain the noodles, then snip them into 2.5 cm (1 inch) lengths. Set the noodles aside.

3 Purée the soup in a food processor or blender. Return it to the rinsed saucepan and add the noodles. Stir in a little chicken stock if necessary. Add the chopped coriander, with salt and pepper to taste. Heat through, then serve.

Pumpkin and lemon soup

alcohol free ✓ | citrus free ✗ | dairy free ✗ | gluten free ✓ | wheat free ✓

Serves 6
Preparation time: 15 minutes
Cooking time: 40 minutes

Per serving
Energy 204 kcals/845 kJ | Protein 3 g | Carbohydrate 13 g | Fat 16 g
Saturated fat 10 g | Fibre 2 g

25 g (1 oz) butter
1 large onion, sliced
500 g (1 lb) pumpkin, peeled, deseeded and cut into chunks
250 g (8 oz) potatoes, sliced
1 small garlic clove, crushed
1 thyme sprig, plus extra to garnish
1.2 litres (2 pints) chicken stock
juice of 1 lemon
150 ml (¼ pint) double cream
salt and pepper

1 Heat the butter in a large heavy saucepan, add the onion and cook over a gentle heat until soft and transparent. Add the pumpkin, potatoes, garlic and thyme. Cover the pan and cook slowly for 20 minutes, or until the vegetables are soft.

2 Pour in the stock, with salt and pepper to taste. Bring to the boil and simmer for 10 minutes. Remove and discard the thyme sprig.

3 Purée the soup in a food processor or blender or rub through a sieve. Squeeze in the lemon juice. Stir in the cream and reheat without boiling. Serve garnished with a thyme sprig.

Chilled fresh fruit soup

alcohol free ✓ | citrus free ✕ | dairy free ✓ | gluten free ✓ | wheat free ✓

Serves 6
Preparation time: 10 minutes, plus chilling

Per serving
Energy 293 kcals/1240 kJ | Protein 3 g | Carbohydrate 73 g | Fat 1 g
Saturated fat 0 g | Fibre 6 g

2 dessert apples, peeled, quartered and cored
6 bananas, roughly chopped
500 g (1 lb) strawberries
375 g (12 oz) pears, peeled, quartered and cored
1 litre (1¾ pints) fresh orange juice
2 tablespoons fresh lemon juice
300 ml (½ pint) fresh grapefruit juice
5–6 tablespoons clear honey
mint sprigs or strawberries, to garnish

1 Place all the fruit in a food processor or blender with 300 ml (½ pint) of the orange juice and blend until very smooth. Add the lemon juice, grapefruit juice and honey. Blend again, in batches if necessary, until the mixture is smooth.

2 Pour the soup into a large bowl, stir in the remaining orange juice and cover the bowl loosely. Chill in the refrigerator for 3–4 hours.

3 Pour the chilled soup into 6 chilled bowls and garnish each one with a mint sprig or a strawberrry.

Japanese miso soup with tofu

alcohol free ✓ | citrus free ✓ | dairy free ✓ | gluten free ✓ | wheat free ✓

Serves 4
Preparation time: 15 minutes
Cooking time: about 45 minutes

Per serving
Energy 52 kcals/216 kJ | Protein 6 g | Carbohydrate 2 g | Fat 2 g
Saturated fat 0 g | Fibre 1 g

2 tablespoons red or white miso
1 small leek
125 g (4 oz) firm tofu
1 tablespoon wakame seaweed

Dashi Stock:
15 g (1½ oz) kombu seaweed
1.8 litres (3 pints) water
2 tablespoons dried tuna (bonito) flakes

To Serve:
bunch of chives
pepper

1 First make the dashi. Wipe the kombu seaweed with a damp cloth and put it into a saucepan with the water. Bring to a simmer, skimming away any scum that rises to the surface. When the soup is clear, add 1½ tablespoons of the dried tuna flakes and simmer, uncovered, for 20 minutes. Remove the pan from the heat and add the remaining dried tuna flakes. Set aside for 5 minutes, then strain the dashi and return to the pan.

2 Mix the miso with a little of the warm stock and add 1 tablespoon at a time to the remaining stock, stirring constantly until the miso has dissolved. Remove from the heat until ready to serve.

3 Cut the leek into fine julienne strips and the tofu into small squares. Warm the miso soup and add the leek and tofu with the wakame seaweed.

4 Blanch the chives, tie into a bundle and float on top of the soup and sprinkle with pepper. Serve immediately.

Haddock and fennel soup

alcohol free ✓ I citrus free ✓ I dairy free ✕ I gluten free ✓ I wheat free ✓

Serves 4
Preparation time: 15 minutes
Cooking time: 25–30 minutes

Per serving
Energy 208 kcals/870 kJ I Protein 15 g I Carbohydrate 18 g I Fat 9 g
Saturated fat 5 g I Fibre 2 g

25 g (1 oz) butter or margarine
250 g (8 oz) fennel bulbs, thinly sliced, leaves reserved for garnish
1 leek, white part only, trimmed, cleaned and sliced
600 ml (1 pint) fish stock
1 bay leaf
300 g (10 oz) potatoes, thinly sliced
250 g (8 oz) haddock fillets, skinned
300 ml (½ pint) milk
½ teaspoon white pepper
salt

1 Melt the butter or margarine in a saucepan. Add the fennel and
leek slices and simmer for 5 minutes or until soft. Add the stock,
bay leaf and potatoes. Bring to the boil, then simmer, covered,
for 10–15 minutes or until tender. Discard the bay leaf.

2 In another saucepan, combine the haddock, milk and white
pepper. Bring to the boil, then simmer, covered, for 5 minutes.
Leave to stand for 5 minutes, then break the fish into flakes.

3 Purée 300 ml (½ pint) of the fennel mixture in a food processor
or blender. Return the purée to the saucepan and add the milk
and fish mixture. Stir well and heat thoroughly without boiling.
Serve garnished with the reserved finely chopped fennel leaves.

Chinese crab soup

alcohol free ✗ | citrus free ✓ | dairy free ✓ | gluten free ✓ | wheat free ✓

Serves 4
Preparation time: 10 minutes
Cooking time: about 20 minutes

Per serving
Energy 90 kcals/380 kJ | Protein 8 g | Carbohydrate 9 g | Fat 2 g
Saturated fat 0 g | Fibre 1 g

1 litre (1¾ pints) chicken stock
2.5 cm (1 inch) piece of root ginger, very finely chopped
2 ripe tomatoes, skinned, deseeded and very finely chopped
½ small red or green chilli, deseeded and very finely chopped
2 tablespoons Chinese rice wine or dry sherry
1 tablespoon rice wine vinegar or white wine or cider vinegar
½ teaspoon sugar
1 tablespoon cornflour
about 150 g (5 oz) white crab meat, defrosted and drained
   thoroughly if frozen
salt and pepper
2 thinly sliced spring onions, to garnish

1 Put the stock into a large saucepan with the ginger, tomatoes,
chilli, rice wine or sherry, vinegar and sugar. Bring to the boil,
cover the pan and simmer for about 10 minutes.

2 Blend the cornflour to a paste with a little cold water, then pour
it into the soup and stir to mix. Simmer, stirring, for 12 minutes
until the soup thickens.

3 Add the crab meat, stir gently to mix, then heat through for 2–3
minutes. Taste the soup and add salt and pepper if necessary.
Serve piping hot, sprinkled with the sliced spring onions.

Lobster and corn chowder

alcohol free ✓ | citrus free ✓ | dairy free ✗ | gluten free ✓ | wheat free ✓

Serves 4
Preparation time: 40 minutes (if preparing the lobster yourself)
Cooking time: about 1 hour

Per serving
Energy 647 kcals/2727 kJ | Protein 43 g | Carbohydrate 67 g | Fat 24 g
Saturated fat 11 g | Fibre 8 g

2 lobsters, 750 g (1½ lb) each
25 g (1 oz) butter
1 onion, finely chopped
1 carrot, finely chopped
1 celery stick, finely chopped
1 thyme sprig
1 parsley sprig
2 bay leaves
1 litre (1¾ pints) water

Chowder:
200 g (7 oz) canned sweetcorn kernels, drained
25 g (1 oz) butter
1 small onion, chopped
1 small garlic clove, crushed
50 g (2 oz) streaky bacon, cut into small strips
300 ml (½ pint) semi-skimmed milk
150 ml (¼ pint) single cream
1 kg (2 lb) potatoes, cut into 1.5 cm (¾ inch) cubes
pinch of cayenne pepper
4 tomatoes, skinned, deseeded and chopped
salt and pepper

1 Cut the lobsters in half lengthways, remove and discard the green tomalley, gills and intestinal vein running along the back. Smash the claws, remove the meat and set aside. Cut the remaining meat into small pieces and set aside. Place the shells in a plastic bag and, using a rolling pin, smash into small pieces.

2 Melt the butter in a large saucepan over a low heat, add the onion, carrot and celery and cook, without colouring, for 8–10 minutes until softened. Add the herbs, water and the broken shells. Bring to the boil, then reduce the heat and simmer for 30 minutes. Strain through a fine sieve into a bowl.

3 To make the chowder, set aside one-third of the corn kernels. Place the remaining corn kernels in a food processor with the lobster broth and blend until smooth.

4 Melt the butter in a large flameproof casserole, add the onion and garlic and cook gently, without colouring, for 5 minutes. Add the bacon and cook until lightly golden.

5 Add the corn purée, milk, cream, potatoes and reserved corn. Bring to the boil, then reduce the heat and simmer for 10–15 minutes. Season to taste with salt, pepper and cayenne. Stir in the tomatoes and lobster meat and heat through gently.

Mulligatawny soup

alcohol free ✓ | citrus free ✓ | dairy free ✗ | gluten free ✓ | wheat free ✓

Serves 6
Preparation time: 25 minutes
Cooking time: 30–40 minutes

Per serving
Energy 317 kcals/1333 kJ | Protein 22 g | Carbohydrate 33 g | Fat 12 g
Saturated fat 3 g | Fibre 4 g

2 garlic cloves, finely chopped
2.5 cm (1 inch) piece of root ginger
1 onion, roughly chopped
25 g (1 oz) butter
2 tablespoons vegetable oil
1 tablespoon ground turmeric
2 teaspoons ground coriander
1 tablespoon Madras curry paste or powder
175 g (6 oz) red lentils
75 g (3 oz) long-grain rice
1.8 litres (3 pints) chicken stock
1 green dessert apple, chopped
2 chicken breasts, cooked and shredded

To Garnish:
oil, for frying
2 onions, thinly sliced
6 tablespoons natural yogurt
1 large green chilli, sliced

1 Place the garlic, ginger and onion in a food processor or blender and process for 1–2 minutes, or until finely chopped.

2 Heat the butter and oil in a large heavy pan over a moderate heat. Add the processed garlic mixture, turmeric, coriander and curry paste or powder. Cook for 4–5 minutes, stirring occasionally, until the onion is brown. Add the lentils and rice and stir to combine. Cook for 2–3 minutes.

3 Add the stock and chopped apple to the pan and stir gently to combine. Bring slowly to the boil and boil for 3 minutes, then reduce the heat and simmer for 20 minutes, or until the lentils and rice are tender. Stir in the chicken, cover and cook for 3 minutes.

4 To make the garnish, heat the oil. Separate the onions into rings and shallow-fry in small batches over a moderate heat until brown and crisp. Drain on kitchen paper.

5 Serve the soup in individual bowls, topped with a spoonful of yogurt and garnished with onion rings and a few chilli slices.

Raindrop soup

alcohol free ✗ | citrus free ✓ | dairy free ✓ | gluten free ✓ | wheat free ✓

Serves 4
Preparation time: 5 minutes
Cooking time: 10 minutes

Per serving
Energy 64 kcals/268 kJ | Protein 8 g | Carbohydrate 7 g | Fat 1 g
Saturated fat 0 g | Fibre 0 g

1 litre (1¾ pints) chicken stock
2 tablespoons Chinese rice wine or dry sherry
200 g (7 oz) canned water chestnuts, drained and very thinly sliced
   into rounds
4 spring onions (white part only), very thinly sliced into rings
125 g (4 oz) cooked peeled prawns
salt and pepper
a few drops of sesame oil, to finish

1 Pour the stock into a large saucepan and bring to the boil over a
high heat. Stir in the rice wine or sherry, then add the water
chestnuts and spring onions and simmer for 2 minutes.

2 Turn the heat down to low and add the prawns. Heat through
gently for 1–2 minutes, then taste and add salt and pepper if
necessary. Stir in a few drops of sesame oil before serving.

Chilled stuffed artichokes

alcohol free ✓ | citrus free ✗ | dairy free ✓ | gluten free ✓ | wheat free ✓

Serves 4
Preparation time: 30 minutes
Cooking time: about 35 minutes

Per serving
Energy 193 kcals/809 kJ | Protein 12 g | Carbohydrate 28 g | Fat 4 g
Saturated fat 1 g | Fibre 1 g

4 artichokes, stems trimmed and top third of leaves removed
1 tablespoon fresh lemon juice
½ quantity Steamed Vegetables with Ginger (see page 190), chilled

Sauce:
150 g (5 oz) tofu, drained
4 tablespoons tomato purée
4 tablespoons horseradish sauce
2 teaspoons fresh lemon juice
2 teaspoons white vinegar
¼ teaspoon grated lemon rind
½ teaspoon onion salt
½ teaspoon sugar
few drops of Tabasco sauce
freshly ground white pepper, to taste

1 Place the artichokes and lemon juice in a deep saucepan and add
boiling water to cover. Cover and cook for 30 minutes, or until
one of the outer artichoke leaves pulls off easily. Remove from
the pan, turn upside down to drain, then refrigerate to cool.

2 Remove the central choke of each artichoke and fill with chilled
vegetables. To make the sauce, purée all the ingredients in a food
processor or blender and pour over each artichoke to serve.

Tempura

alcohol free ✗ | citrus free ✓ | dairy free ✓ | gluten free ✗ | wheat free ✗

Serves 4
Preparation time: 30 minutes
Cooking time: 20–30 minutes

Per serving
Energy 483 kcals/2029 kJ | Protein 35 g | Carbohydrate 48 g | Fat 16 g
Saturated fat 2 g | Fibre 5 g

900 ml (1½ pints) oil, for deep-frying
12 raw tiger prawns, peeled, but with tails left on
500 g (1 lb) plaice or sole fillets, skinned and cut into small pieces
8 button mushrooms
1 bunch of spring onions, cut into 3.5 cm (1½ inch) lengths
1 red pepper, cored, deseeded and sliced
1 green pepper, cored, deseeded and sliced
1 large onion, cut into wedges
½ small cauliflower, broken into florets
½ small aubergine, thinly sliced
chives, to garnish

Batter:
1 egg
150 ml (¼ pint) water
125 g (4 oz) plain flour
50 g (2 oz) cornflour
pinch of salt

Dipping Sauce:
300 ml (½ pint) canned chicken consommé
4 tablespoons sweet vermouth or sherry
4 tablespoons light soy sauce

1 To make the batter, lightly beat the egg in a large bowl. Beat in the water until frothy. Sift together the flour, cornflour and salt and fold in gradually.

2 Heat the oil in a wok. Dip the prawns, fish pieces and vegetables into the batter, then deep-fry in batches, until golden. Drain on kitchen paper; keep warm.

3 To make the dipping sauce, gently heat all the ingredients in a saucepan, then transfer to a warmed bowl. Serve immediately.

Baked stuffed mushrooms

alcohol free ✓ | citrus free ✓ | dairy free ✕ | gluten free ✕ | wheat free ✕

Serves 4
Preparation time: 10 minutes
Cooking time: 25 minutes

Per serving
Energy 166 kcals/692 kJ | Protein 6 g | Carbohydrate 11 g | Fat 11 g
Saturated fat 3 g | Fibre 2 g

4 large field mushrooms
1 small onion, very finely chopped
50 g (2 oz) mini macaroni, cooked
25 g (1 oz) walnuts, chopped
1 tablespoon chopped parsley
25 g (1 oz) Cheddar cheese, cubed
1 tablespoon tomato purée
1 egg, beaten
1 tablespoon olive oil
salt and pepper

1 Chop the mushroom stalks finely and set aside. Peel the
mushrooms, if blemished, and grill for 5 minutes until just
softened. Remove and set aside.

2 Put the chopped onion into a large bowl. Add the chopped
mushroom stalks, cooked macaroni, walnuts, parsley, cheese and
tomato purée. Mix well, then add enough of the beaten egg to
bind the mixture. Add salt and pepper to taste.

3 Divide the filling between the mushrooms and drizzle over a
little olive oil. Place well apart on a grill pan.

4 Grill for 15–20 minutes until the top of the stuffing is crisp and
has started to char at the edges.

Fish and seafood

Sea bass with fennel

alcohol free ✓ | citrus free ✓ | dairy free ✓ | gluten free ✓ | wheat free ✓

Serves 4
Preparation time: 5 minutes
Cooking time: 45–50 minutes

Per serving
Energy 384 kcals/1600 kJ | Protein 44 g | Carbohydrate 2 g | Fat 22 g
Saturated fat 3 g | Fibre 2 g

2 large fennel bulbs
6 tablespoons olive oil
8 tablespoons water
2 sea bass, about 500 g (1 lb) each, filleted
salt and pepper

1 Cut the fennel bulbs lengthways into 1 cm (½ inch) slices. Pour
the oil into a wok, add the fennel and water and bring to the
boil. Cover and simmer for 30 minutes, until the fennel is very
tender, stirring occasionally.

2 Remove the lid, season the fennel with salt and pepper and boil
until all the water has evaporated and the fennel is golden
brown. Transfer to a warmed plate and keep hot.

3 Season the fish with salt and pepper, add to the wok and baste
with the hot oil. Cover and cook for 7–8 minutes. Turn the fish
over, baste again and cook for about 5 more minutes.

4 Arrange the fennel on a warmed serving dish, place the fish on
the fennel and pour the cooking juices around and over the fish.

Steamed spiced fish

alcohol free ✓ | citrus free ✗ | dairy free ✓ | gluten free ✓ | wheat free ✓

Serves 6
Preparation time: 10 minutes, plus standing
Cooking time: 15–20 minutes

Per serving
Energy 210 kcals/880 kJ | Protein 33 g | Carbohydrate 1 g | Fat 8 g
Saturated fat 1 g | Fibre 0 g

1.5 kg (3 lb) whole bass, bream or grey mullet, cleaned
1 tablespoon sea salt
1 tablespoon cumin seeds, lightly crushed
5 cm (2 inch) piece of root ginger, finely chopped
2 tablespoons fresh lemon juice
2 tablespoons olive oil
2–3 garlic cloves, finely chopped
1 tablespoon coriander seeds, crushed
spring onion curls, to garnish
pepper

1 Rinse the fish in cold water, then rub it all over with salt and lots of black pepper. Leave to stand, covered, at room temperature for 30 minutes.

2 Put a grill rack into a roasting pan and pour in 2.5 cm (1 inch) boiling water. Set over a low heat so the liquid is gently simmering.

3 Transfer the fish to a heatproof serving plate, discarding any liquid which may have collected around it. Sprinkle on the cumin seeds and ginger, then put the plate on to the rack. Cover the whole roasting pan with foil, pressing it around the edges to form as close a seal as possible, then cook for 15–20 minutes until the fish flakes easily. Test it with the point of a sharp knife near the gills. Take off the heat, remove the foil, and sprinkle over the lemon juice.

4 Heat the oil in a small frying pan. Stir-fry the garlic and coriander seeds over a high heat for about 1 minute. Pour the sizzling oil over the fish, garnish with spring onion curls and serve.

Japanese tofu and fish hotpot

alcohol free ✓ | citrus free ✓ | dairy free ✓ | gluten free ✕ | wheat free ✕

Serves 6
Preparation time: 30 minutes, plus soaking
Cooking time: about 30 minutes

Per serving
Energy 406 kcals/1699 kJ | Protein 35 g | Carbohydrate 44 g | Fat 9 g
Saturated fat 2 g | Fibre 1 g

6 Chinese cabbage leaves
125 g (4 oz) sugar snap peas
300 g (10 oz) cellophane noodles (saifan)
2 boneless, skinless chicken thighs
125 g (4 oz) sea bream fillets
125 g (4 oz) mackerel fillets
1.8 litres (3 pints) fish stock
5 tablespoons mirin (sweet Japanese rice wine)
2.5 cm (1 inch) piece of root ginger, grated
6 spring onions, chopped
1 tablespoon soy sauce
175 g (6 oz) clams
125 g (4 oz) small cooked, peeled prawns
250 g (8 oz) firm tofu, cubed
75 g (3 oz) watercress, chopped
125 g (4 oz) enoki or shiitake mushrooms, halved

Red Maple Relish:
75 g (3 oz) daikon radish
2 small chillies

1 Blanch the cabbage and sugar snap peas in boiling water for 1 minute, then drain and refresh in cold water. Shred the cabbage.

2 Place the noodles in a large bowl, cover with hot water and leave to soak for about 10 minutes or until softened.

3 Slice the chicken into cubes and the fish into 5 cm (2 inch) pieces. Put the stock, mirin, ginger, spring onions and soy sauce into a large pan and bring to the boil. Reduce the heat to a simmer, add the chicken and simmer for 8–10 minutes.

4 To make the red maple relish, make two deep holes in the large end of the daikon with a chopstick and insert the chillies. Grate the daikon and chillies together very finely. Then put them in a mortar and pound with a pestle.

5 Add the clams, prawns, sliced fish, soaked noodles and tofu to the simmering hotpot. Simmer for a further 6–8 minutes or until the clams open and the fish has cooked. Discard any clams that remain closed.

6 Arrange the cabbage, blanched sugar snap peas, watercress, mushrooms and red maple relish on a serving platter and serve with the hotpot. Add the watercress and mushrooms to the hotpot and cook for 1 minute. Place a few items in each serving bowl and ladle some stock over the top. Allow diners to help themselves to more as they eat.

Halibut on a bed of vegetables

alcohol free ✓ | citrus free ✓ | dairy free ✗ | gluten free ✓ | wheat free ✓

Serves 2
Preparation time: 20 minutes
Cooking time: about 25 minutes

Per serving
Energy 382 kcals/1594 kJ | Protein 30 g | Carbohydrate 9 g | Fat 26 g
Saturated fat 4 g | Fibre 4 g

2 tablespoons olive oil
½ red pepper, cored, deseeded and roughly chopped
½ green pepper, cored, deseeded and roughly chopped
50 g (2 oz) mushrooms, sliced
1 courgette, sliced lengthways into 3 cm (1½ inch) pieces
½ aubergine, sliced lengthways into 3 cm (1½ inch) pieces
2 tomatoes, skinned and chopped
1 tablespoon tomato purée
2 halibut steaks, about 150–175 g (5–6 oz) each
25 g (1 oz) butter
2 tablespoons chopped mixed parsley, tarragon and chives
salt and pepper

1 Heat the oil in a large saucepan, add the red and green peppers, mushrooms, courgette, aubergine, tomatoes and tomato purée and fry for 15–20 minutes over a moderate heat, stirring occasionally.

2 Meanwhile, line a baking sheet with a large piece of foil, allowing sufficient to fold over comfortably. Place the fish on the foil, dot with butter, sprinkle with 1 tablespoon of the herbs and season with salt and pepper. Fold the foil loosely over the fish and bake in a preheated oven, 200°C (400°F), Gas Mark 6, for 18–20 minutes until cooked through.

3 When the fish and vegetables are cooked, season to taste and add more herbs or tomato purée if necessary. Spoon the vegetables on to warmed plates and put the halibut on top. Serve immediately, sprinkled with the remaining herbs.

Smoked haddock with red pepper sauce

alcohol free ✓ | citrus free ✓ | dairy free ✗ | gluten free ✓ | wheat free ✓

Serves 2
Preparation time: 10 minutes
Cooking time: about 25 minutes

Per serving
Energy 373 kcals/1568 kJ | Protein 42 g | Carbohydrate 19 g | Fat 15 g
Saturated fat 2 g | Fibre 2 g

2 smoked haddock fillets
300 ml (½ pint) semi-skimmed milk
1 tablespoon olive oil
2 shallots, finely chopped
1 garlic clove, crushed
2 large red peppers, cored, deseeded, and finely chopped
200 ml (7 fl oz) half-fat crème fraîche
1 tablespoon chopped tarragon, plus extra to garnish
salt and pepper

1 Put the haddock fillets into a shallow pan, add the milk and poach for 5 minutes, or until done. Remove the haddock, cover and keep warm. Strain and reserve the milk.

2 Meanwhile, heat the oil in a frying pan, add the shallots and garlic and fry gently for 5 minutes until soft. Add the red peppers and cook gently for 7–8 minutes, stirring occasionally.

3 Put the crème fraĉche into a bowl and stir in 4 tablespoons of the strained milk. Stir in the red pepper mixture (or purée it in a food processor if you would like a very smooth sauce). Return the mixture to the pan and add the tarragon. Season the sauce to taste with salt and pepper, then simmer for 10 minutes.

4 To serve, pour the sauce on to the plate and place the haddock on top of the sauce. Sprinkle with pepper, garnish with tarragon and serve immediately.

Cod baked with potatoes, onions and tomatoes

alcohol free ✗ | citrus free ✓ | dairy free ✗ | gluten free ✗ | wheat free ✗

Serves 4
Preparation time: 15 minutes
Cooking time: about 30 minutes

Per serving
Energy 430 kcals/1813 kJ | Protein 36 g | Carbohydrate 33 g | Fat 16 g
 Saturated fat 4 g | Fibre 4 g

12 small new potatoes
1 tablespoon olive oil
4 cod fillets
2 tablespoons extra virgin olive oil
2 onions, finely chopped
1 garlic clove, crushed
1 tablespoon chopped oregano
425 g (14 oz) can chopped tomatoes
125 ml (4 fl oz) dry white wine or fish stock
75 g (3 oz) fine breadcrumbs
50 g (2 oz) grated Parmesan or Cheddar cheese
salt and pepper
chopped parsley, to garnish

1 Boil the potatoes until almost done. Cut them into thick slices and coat in olive oil. Arrange them around a greased ovenproof dish and place the fish in the centre.

2 Meanwhile, heat the extra virgin olive oil in a pan, add the onions and sauté for about 5 minutes until soft. Add the garlic and oregano and cook for 2–3 minutes. Add the tomatoes, wine or stock and salt and pepper to taste and simmer for a few minutes.

3 Spoon half of the tomato mixture over the potatoes and fish. Mix the remaining mixture with the breadcrumbs and cheese and then pour over the fish. Bake in a preheated oven, 200°C (400°F), Gas Mark 6, for 15 minutes or until the fish is cooked. Garnish with parsley.

Sauté of scallops with mangetout

alcohol free ✓ | citrus free ✓ | dairy free ✓ | gluten free ✗ | wheat free ✗

Serves 2
Preparation time: 15 minutes
Cooking time: about 10 minutes

Per serving
Energy 344 kcals/1438 kJ | Protein 24 g | Carbohydrate 11 g | Fat 23 g
Saturated fat 3 g | Fibre 4 g

8 shelled scallops with coral
3 tablespoons vegetable oil
6 spring onions, thinly sliced diagonally
2.5 cm (1 inch) piece of root ginger, finely chopped
175 g (6 oz) mangetout, trimmed
1 garlic clove, crushed
1 tablespoon sesame oil
2 tablespoons soy sauce
½ teaspoon caster sugar
pepper
spring onions, to garnish

1 Slice the scallops thickly, detaching the corals and keeping them whole. Set the corals aside.

2 Heat 2 tablespoons of the vegetable oil in a wok over a moderate heat. Add the spring onions and ginger and stir-fry for a few seconds. Add the mangetout and garlic and stir-fry for 2 minutes, then tip the vegetable mixture into a bowl and set aside.

3 Heat the remaining vegetable oil with the sesame seed oil over a moderate heat. Add the sliced scallops and stir-fry for 3 minutes. Return the spring onion, ginger and mangetout mixture to the wok, add the reserved corals, soy sauce and sugar and increase the heat to high. Toss for 1–2 minutes or until all the ingredients are combined and piping hot. Season with pepper to taste and serve immediately, garnished with spring onions.

Steamed masala mussels

alcohol free ✓ | citrus free ✗ | dairy free ✓ | gluten free ✓ | wheat free ✓

Serves 4
Preparation time: about 40 minutes
Cooking time: 10–15 minutes

Per serving
Energy 211 kcals/886 kJ | Protein 21 g | Carbohydrate 7 g | Fat 11 g
Saturated fat 2 g | Fibre 1 g

3 tablespoons groundnut oil
2 red onions, very finely chopped
4 garlic cloves, crushed
2 tablespoons grated root ginger
3 large green chillies, deseeded and finely chopped
¼ teaspoon saffron threads (optional), infused in 2 tablespoons
    boiling water for 10 minutes
2 teaspoons ground coriander
2 teaspoons ground cumin
1.5 kg (3 lb) mussels, scrubbed and debearded
½ teaspoon salt
300 ml (½ pint) water
2 tablespoons fresh lime juice
4 tablespoons chopped coriander
a few coriander sprigs, to garnish (optional)

1 Heat the oil in a large deep saucepan, add the onions, garlic, ginger and chillies and cook over a gentle heat, stirring occasionally, for 5 minutes or until softened. Stir in the saffron, if using, with its infusing water, or add 2 tablespoons of plain water. Add the ground coriander and cumin and cook for 1 further minute.

2 Add the salt and water to the pan, then stir in the mussels. Cover the pan and cook for about 5–6 minutes or until all the mussels have opened and cooked through. Discard any mussels that have not opened. Stir the lime juice and chopped coriander into the pan; taste and adjust the seasoning if necessary.

3 Ladle the hot mussels and the masala sauce into bowls and garnish with coriander, if liked. Serve immediately.

Stir-fried prawn supper

alcohol free ✓ I citrus free ✓ I dairy free ✓ I gluten free ✕ I wheat free ✕

Serves 4
Preparation time: 10 minutes
Cooking time: 5–7 minutes

Per serving
Energy 380 kcals/1595 kJ I Protein 49 g I Carbohydrate 15 g I Fat 14 g
Saturated fat 2 g I Fibre 5 g

4 tablespoons vegetable oil
1 cm (½ inch) piece of root ginger, peeled and finely sliced into
   matchsticks
2 garlic cloves, chopped
8 spring onions, trimmed and sliced diagonally
1 carrot, peeled and cut into matchsticks
8 celery sticks, sliced diagonally
375 g (12 oz) cauliflower, separated into tiny florets
2 red peppers, cored, deseeded and sliced
1 green pepper, cored, deseeded and sliced
1 kg (2 lb) large raw peeled prawns
celery leaves, to garnish

Glaze:
2 teaspoons cornflour
6 tablespoons water
2 tablespoons white wine vinegar
2 teaspoons soy sauce
2 teaspoons tomato purée
salt and pepper

1 Heat the oil in a wok or deep frying pan, add the ginger and garlic and stir-fry over a moderate heat for 30 seconds. Add the spring onions, carrot and celery and stir-fry for 1 minute, then add the cauliflower and stir-fry for 30 seconds. Add the red and green peppers and stir-fry for a further 30 seconds. Add the prawns and cook for 2–3 minutes.

2 Mix together all the ingredients for the glaze, pour into the pan and stir over a brisk heat until all the prawns and vegetables are coated. Turn on to warmed plates, garnish with the celery leaves and serve immediately.

Stir-fried prawns with tofu

alcohol free ✕ | citrus free ✕ | dairy free ✓ | gluten free ✕ | wheat free ✕

Serves 3
Preparation time: 10 minutes
Cooking time: about 10 minutes

Per serving
Energy 317 kcals/1322 kJ | Protein 27 g | Carbohydrate 9 g | Fat 20 g
Saturated fat 4 g | Fibre 0 g

about 300 ml (½ pint) groundnut oil, for frying
250 g (8 oz) firm tofu, drained, dried and cut into cubes
250 g (8 oz) cooked peeled prawns, defrosted and dried thoroughly
   if frozen

Sauce:
2 tablespoons soy sauce
2 tablespoons Chinese rice wine or dry sherry
1 tablespoon lemon juice
1 teaspoon caster sugar
2 teaspoons cornflour
100 ml (3½ fl oz) cold fish stock or water

1 First prepare the sauce. Put the soy sauce, rice wine or sherry and the lemon juice into a bowl or jug, add the sugar and cornflour and stir well to mix. Stir in the stock or water. Set aside.

2 Heat the oil in a wok until very hot but not smoking. Add the tofu and shallow-fry for 2–3 minutes or until it is golden on all sides, taking care not to let it break up. Lift out with a slotted spoon, drain on kitchen paper and keep warm.

3 Very carefully pour off all but about 1 tablespoon of oil from the wok. Add the prawns, increase the heat to high and stir-fry for 1–2 minutes. Stir the sauce to mix, then pour it into the wok. Bring to the boil, stirring, then add the tofu and stir gently to mix with the prawns and coat in the sauce. Serve immediately.

Chicken dishes

Cranberry chicken stir-fry with ginger

alcohol free ✓ | citrus free ✓ | dairy free ✓ | gluten free ✗ | wheat free ✗

Serves 4
Preparation time: 20 minutes
Cooking time: 10 minutes

Per serving
Energy 228 kcals/957 kJ | Protein 29 g | Carbohydrate 7 g | Fat 10 g
Saturated fat 2 g | Fibre 3 g

2 tablespoons vegetable oil
2 shallots, finely chopped
2.5 cm (1 inch) piece of root ginger, thinly sliced into matchsticks
2 garlic cloves, crushed
4 boneless, skinless chicken breasts, thinly sliced
2 tablespoons hoisin sauce or dark soy sauce
2 tablespoons oyster sauce (optional)
1 tablespoon light soy sauce
25 g (1 oz) dried cranberries
4 spring onions, diagonally sliced
175 g (6 oz) bean sprouts, or sliced green or red pepper
    or carrot strips

To Garnish:
vegetable oil, for deep-frying
handful of basil leaves
1 large red chilli, deseeded and thinly sliced

1 Heat the oil in a wok and stir-fry the shallots, ginger and garlic for 30 seconds. Add the chicken and stir-fry for 2 minutes or until golden brown.

2 Add the hoisin, oyster and soy sauces and the cranberries and stir-fry for a further 2 minutes. Check that the chicken is cooked all the way through, then add the spring onions and bean sprouts or other vegetables and stir-fry for 4 minutes. Transfer to a warmed dish.

3 To make the garnish, heat 1 cm (½ inch) oil in a small saucepan and deep-fry the basil leaves and red chilli in batches for 10–30 seconds until crisp. Remove with a slotted spoon and drain on kitchen paper, then sprinkle over the chicken.

Sichuan bang bang chicken

alcohol free ✗ | citrus free ✓ | dairy free ✓ | gluten free ✗ | wheat free ✗

Serves 4
Preparation time: about 30 minutes, plus cooling
Cooking time: about 15 minutes

Per serving
Energy 419 kcals/1755 kJ | Protein 37 g | Carbohydrate 18 g | Fat 23 g
Saturated fat 4 g | Fibre 4 g

4 boneless, skinless chicken breasts
6 tablespoons soy sauce
2 tablespoons sesame oil
2.5 cm (1 inch) piece of root ginger, peeled and finely chopped
2 tablespoons sesame seeds
4 tablespoons vegetable oil
4 carrots, cut into julienne strips
1 fresh green or red chilli, deseeded and chopped
125 g (4 oz) bean sprouts
½ cucumber, cut into julienne strips
3 tablespoons Chinese rice wine or dry sherry
2 tablespoons clear honey
150 ml (¼ pint) chicken stock
flat leaf parsley, to garnish

1 Place the chicken between 2 sheets of greaseproof paper and pound with the bottom of a saucepan to flatten. Cut the chicken into thin strips across the grain, then place in a shallow dish. Mix 2 tablespoons of the soy sauce with the sesame oil and ginger. Pour over the chicken and turn to coat. Cover and leave to marinate for 20 minutes, turning occasionally.

2 Meanwhile, heat the wok until hot. Add the sesame seeds and dry-fry over a gentle heat for 1–2 minutes or until toasted, tossing so they do not burn. Remove the wok from the heat and tip the seeds on to a plate. Set aside.

3 Return the wok to a moderate heat with 2 tablespoons of the vegetable oil. Add the carrots and chilli and stir-fry for 2–3 minutes. Remove with a slotted spoon and place in a bowl. Add the bean sprouts to the wok and stir-fry for 1 minute, then tip the bean sprouts into the bowl. Add the cucumber strips to the bowl and toss well.

4 Heat the remaining oil in the wok. Add the chicken, increase the heat and stir-fry for 4–5 minutes. Transfer the chicken to a separate bowl. Add the remaining soy sauce, the rice wine or sherry, honey and stock to the wok. Bring to the boil, stirring, then simmer for a few minutes, stirring constantly, until reduced slightly. Pour half of the sauce mixture over the vegetables and half over the chicken. Stir to mix, then cover and leave to cool, stirring occasionally.

5 Arrange the chicken and vegetables on individual plates, drizzle over any remaining sauce and sprinkle with the sesame seeds. Garnish with parsley and serve.

Thai minced chicken with basil

alcohol free ✓ | citrus free ✓ | dairy free ✓ | gluten free ✕ | wheat free ✕

Serves 2
Preparation time: 6 minutes
Cooking time: 6 minutes

Per serving
Energy 399 kcals/1653 kJ | Protein 19 g | Carbohydrate 14 g | Fat 30 g
Saturated fat 5 g | Fibre 1 g

5 small green chillies
2 garlic cloves
2 tablespoons oil
125 g (4 oz) minced chicken
1 shallot, chopped
25 g (1 oz) bamboo shoots
25 g (1 oz) red pepper, cored, deseeded and chopped
15 g (½ oz) carrot, diced
1 teaspoon palm sugar or light muscovado sugar
3 tablespoons Thai fish sauce or light soy sauce
3 tablespoons chicken stock
15 g (½ oz) basil leaves, finely chopped
rice, to serve

Crispy Garlic, Shallot and Basil Garnish:
groundnut oil, for deep-frying
25 g (1 oz) garlic, finely chopped
25 g (1 oz) shallots, finely chopped
25 g (1 oz) basil leaves
1 small red chilli, thinly sliced

1 To make the garnish, heat the oil in a wok. When it is hot, add the garlic and stir for about 40 seconds. Remove with a slotted spoon, draining as much oil as possible back into the wok, then dry on kitchen paper. Repeat the process with the shallots, allowing 1½–2 minutes frying time. Then add the basil leaves and chilli to the oil and fry for about 1 minute. Remove with a slotted spoon and drain as before.

2 To cook the chicken, put the chillies and garlic into a mortar and pound with a pestle until well broken down.

3 Heat the oil in a wok, add the pounded chillies and garlic and stir-fry for 30 seconds. Add the remaining ingredients and cook, stirring, for 4 minutes over a moderate heat. Increase the heat to high and stir vigorously for 30 seconds.

4 Transfer to a warmed dish and serve with rice and sprinkled with the crispy garlic, shallot and basil garnish.

Stir-fried chicken with cashew nuts and baby corn

alcohol free ✓ | citrus free ✓ | dairy free ✓ | gluten free ✗ | wheat free ✗

Serves 2
Preparation time: 10 minutes
Cooking time: about 7 minutes

Per serving
Energy 414 kcals/1726 kJ | Protein 23 g | Carbohydrate 22 g | Fat 26 g
Saturated fat 4 g | Fibre 0 g

2 tablespoons oil
125 g (4 oz) chicken, skinned and cut into bite-sized pieces
¼ onion, sliced
50 g (2 oz) baby corn, diagonally sliced
50 g (2 oz) cashew nuts
125 ml (4 fl oz) light soy sauce
4 tablespoons chicken stock
4 teaspoons palm sugar or light muscovado sugar
15 g (½ oz) spring onion, diagonally sliced
pepper
1 large red chilli, diagonally sliced, to garnish

1 Heat the oil in a wok, add the chicken, onion, baby corn and cashew nuts. Stir-fry over a high heat for 3 minutes.

2 Reduce the heat and stir in the soy sauce, then add the stock, sugar and spring onion and season with pepper. Raise the heat and stir-fry for another 2 minutes.

3 Turn on to a serving dish or into 2 individual bowls, sprinkle with sliced chilli and serve.

Thai green chicken curry

alcohol free ✓ | citrus free ✗ | dairy free ✓ | gluten free ✗ | wheat free ✗

Serves 2
Preparation time: 5–7 minutes
Cooking time: 13–15 minutes

Per serving
Energy 230 kcals/969 kJ | Protein 18 g | Carbohydrate 17 g | Fat 11 g
Saturated fat 1 g | Fibre 2 g

1 tablespoon oil
1½ tablespoons ready-made green curry paste
4 tablespoons coconut milk
125 g (4 oz) chicken breast, cut into bite-sized pieces
2 lime leaves, torn, or 2 strips lime rind
½ lemon grass stalk, cut in fine, oblique slices (optional)
50 g (2 oz) bamboo shoots
3 small green aubergines, or 1 purple aubergine, chopped
50 g (2 oz) courgettes, cut into diagonal chunks
1 large red chilli, diagonally sliced
6 tablespoons chicken stock
1 tablespoon palm sugar or light muscovado sugar
3 tablespoons Thai fish sauce or light soy sauce
basil sprigs, to garnish

1 Heat the oil in a wok and stir in the curry paste. Cook for
30 seconds, then add the coconut milk and cook, stirring, for
1 minute.

2 Add the chicken, bring to a simmer, then add all the remaining
ingredients. Simmer gently for 10 minutes, stirring occasionally.

3 Transfer the curry to a warmed serving bowl, garnish with basil
sprigs and serve.

Chicken with pine nuts

alcohol free ✕ | citrus free ✕ | dairy free ✓ | gluten free ✕ | wheat free ✕

Serves 4
Preparation time: 30 minutes
Cooking time: 15 minutes

Per serving
Energy 438 kcals/1830 kJ | Protein 36 g | Carbohydrate 16 g | Fat 25 g
Saturated fat 3 g | Fibre 1 g

4 boneless, skinless chicken breasts, cut into 1 x 5 cm (½ x 2 inch) strips
4 tablespoons sunflower oil
1 red pepper, cored, deseeded and cut into strips
1 green pepper, cored, deseeded and cut into strips
1 red chilli, deseeded and finely chopped
1 green chilli, deseeded and finely chopped, plus extra to garnish
50 g (2 oz) pine nuts
1 garlic clove, finely chopped
4 tablespoons dry white wine
2 tablespoons fresh lemon juice
3 tablespoons oyster sauce
2 teaspoons caster sugar
1 teaspoon chilli sauce
4 tablespoons light soy sauce
1 tablespoon cornflour
salt and pepper
½ lime, to serve

To Garnish:
2 spring onions, sliced
flat leaf parsley sprigs

1 Season the chicken strips with salt and pepper. Heat 2 tablespoons of oil in a wok, add the chicken strips and cook, stirring constantly, for 5 minutes, or until tender. Remove the chicken and reserve.

2 Heat the remaining oil in the wok and stir-fry the red and green pepper strips for 2 minutes, until just cooked. Lift out and put to one side.

3 Add the chillies, pine nuts and garlic and stir-fry for 1 minute. Drain and discard any excess fat, then add the white wine, lemon juice, oyster sauce, caster sugar and chilli sauce. Cook, stirring, for 1 minute.

4 Blend the soy sauce and cornflour, add to the chilli mixture and bring to the boil. Return the chicken and peppers to the wok, then cover and cook over a moderate heat until warmed through. Serve immediately with the ½ lime and garnished with the spring onions, parsley and green chilli.

Shredded chicken with green peppers

alcohol free ✗ | citrus free ✓ | dairy free ✓ | gluten free ✓ | wheat free ✓

Serves 4
Preparation time: 10–15 minutes
Cooking time: 10 minutes

Per serving
Energy 225 kcals/942 kJ | Protein 18 g | Carbohydrate 9 g | Fat 14 g
Saturated fat 2 g | Fibre 1 g

2 boneless, skinless chicken breasts, cut into thin strips
1½ teaspoons salt
1 egg white, lightly beaten
3 teaspoons cornflour
4 tablespoons oil
1 spring onion, finely chopped
2 slices root ginger, finely chopped
250 g (8 oz) green peppers, cored, deseeded and cut into
    matchsticks
2 tablespoons Chinese rice wine or dry sherry

To Garnish:
1 teaspoon sesame seeds
spring onion strips
lime wedges
sliced red chilli

1 Mix the chicken first with ½ teaspoon of the salt, then the egg white and finally 2 teaspoons of the cornflour. Blend the remaining cornflour in a jug with a little water.

2 Heat a wok until hot. Add the oil and heat, then add the chicken strips and stir-fry over a moderate heat until they turn white, then remove with a slotted spoon and set aside.

3 Increase the heat to high and, when the oil is very hot, add the spring onion and ginger to flavour the oil. Add the green peppers and cook, stirring constantly, for 30 seconds, then return the chicken shreds with the remaining salt and the wine or sherry. Stir-fry for 1 minute, then add the blended cornflour. Mix well. Serve at once garnished with sesame seeds, spring onion strips, lime wedges and sliced red chilli.

Chicken with sizzling garlic sauce

alcohol free ✗ | citrus free ✓ | dairy free ✓ | gluten free ✓ | wheat free ✓

Serves 2
Preparation time: 10–15 minutes, plus marinating
Cooking time: 10 minutes

Per serving
Energy 526 kcals/2207 kJ | Protein 31 g | Carbohydrate 50 g | Fat 24 g
Saturated fat 5 g | Fibre 1 g

2 boneless, skinless chicken breasts, total weight 250–300 g
   (8–10 oz), cut into thin strips
1 small egg
2 garlic cloves, crushed
about 4 tablespoons cornflour
about 175 ml (6 fl oz) groundnut oil, for frying
salt and pepper
a few drops of chilli oil (optional), to serve

Garlic Sauce:
4 spring onions (white part only), finely shredded
2 garlic cloves, finely chopped
200 ml (7 fl oz) hot chicken stock
4 tablespoons Chinese rice wine or dry sherry
1 teaspoon cornflour

To Garnish:
½ tablespoon finely chopped red pepper
½ tablespoon finely chopped green pepper
1 tablespoon chopped coriander (optional)

1 Put the chicken breasts between clingfilm and pound them with the bottom of a saucepan to flatten them. Remove the clingfilm and cut the chicken into strips about 2.5 cm (1 inch) wide.

2 Beat the egg in a bowl with the crushed garlic and plenty of salt and pepper. Dip the chicken strips in the egg mixture, then place them in a single layer on a plate and dredge them with cornflour. Put the plate in the refrigerator for about 1 hour, or longer if you have the time.

3 Heat the oil in a wok until very hot, but not smoking. Immerse the chicken pieces in the hot oil in a single layer. Fry for about 3 minutes or until the chicken is golden, turning once. Remove with a slotted spoon and keep hot in a warmed bowl. Repeat with the remaining chicken.

4 Very carefully pour off all but about 1 teaspoon of the hot oil from the wok. Return the wok to a low heat and make the sauce. Put the spring onions, chopped garlic, stock and rice wine or sherry in the wok. Increase the heat to high and bring to the boil, stirring.

5 Blend the cornflour to a paste with a little cold water, then pour it into the wok and stir to mix. Simmer, stirring, for 1–2 minutes until the sauce thickens, then pour it over the chicken. Garnish with the red and green pepper and chopped coriander, if using, and sprinkle with a few drops of chilli oil, if liked. Serve immediately.

Chicken and prawn kebabs

alcohol free ✓ | citrus free ✗ | dairy free ✓ | gluten free ✓ | wheat free ✓

Serves 6
Preparation time: 15 minutes, plus marinating
Cooking time: about 20 minutes

Per serving
Energy 250 kcals/1053 kJ | Protein 34 g | Carbohydrate 2 g | Fat 12 g
Saturated fat 2 g | Fibre 1 g

750 g (1½ lb) boneless, skinless chicken breasts, cut into 2.5 cm
    (1 inch) cubes
20 cooked large prawns
1 small yellow or red pepper, cored, deseeded and cut into 2.5 cm
    (1 inch) squares
1 small green pepper, cored, deseeded and cut into 2.5 cm (1 inch)
    squares
lime wedges, to garnish

Herb Marinade:
4 tablespoons sunflower oil
2 tablespoons lemon juice
1 teaspoon chopped marjoram
1 teaspoon chopped thyme
2 tablespoons chopped parsley
1 garlic clove, crushed
1 onion, finely chopped
salt and pepper

1 Thread the chicken, prawns and peppers alternately on to presoaked bamboo or oiled metal skewers. Mix together all the ingredients for the herb marinade in a bowl with salt and pepper to taste. Place the skewers in a shallow dish and pour over the marinade. Turn the skewers to coat with the marinade. Cover and leave for 2 hours in a cool place, turning occasionally.

2 Remove the kebabs from the marinade, reserving the marinade. Cook the kebabs under a preheated moderate hot grill for about 20 minutes, turning and basting frequently with the reserved marinade.

3 Serve garnished with lime wedges.

Stir-fried chicken with pineapple

alcohol free ✓ | citrus free ✓ | dairy free ✓ | gluten free ✗ | wheat free ✗

Serves 4
Preparation time: 10 minutes
Cooking time: 12–14 minutes

Per serving
Energy 270 kcals/1136 kJ | Protein 11 g | Carbohydrate 22 g | Fat 16 g
Saturated fat 3 g | Fibre 2 g

oil, for deep-frying
50 g (2 oz) Japanese tempura flour or self-raising flour
75 ml (3 fl oz) water
125 g (4 oz) chicken, skinned and cut into bite-sized pieces
1 tablespoon groundnut oil
150 g (5 oz) fresh pineapple, cut into chunks
1 tomato, cut into 8 pieces
1 tablespoon tomato purée
1 tablespoon palm sugar or light muscovado sugar
50 g (2 oz) cashew nuts
1½ tablespoons light soy sauce

To Garnish:
alfalfa or bean sprouts
coriander sprigs
½ lime

1 Heat the oil for deep-frying in a wok and, while it is heating, mix the flour and water to make a coating batter.

2 When the oil is hot enough, coat half the chicken pieces in the batter and deep-fry them until they are golden brown. Remove them from the oil and drain on kitchen paper. Repeat with the remaining chicken.

3 Pour off the oil, wipe the wok with kitchen paper, then heat the groundnut oil. Add the pineapple, tomato, tomato purée, sugar and cashews and stir-fry for 2 minutes. Add the soy sauce and continue to stir.

4 Serve the batter-coated chicken on the tomato and pineapple mixture, garnished with alfalfa or bean sprouts, coriander sprigs and ½ lime.

Chicken, squash and sweet potato tagine

alcohol free ✓ | citrus free ✓ | dairy free ✓ | gluten free ✓ | wheat free ✓

Serves 4
Preparation time: 20 minutes
Cooking time: 1 hour

Per serving
Energy 465 kcals/1953 kJ | Protein 40 g | Carbohydrate 48 g | Fat 14 g
Saturated fat 3 g | Fibre 8 g

2 tablespoons olive oil
700 g (1½ lb) boneless, skinless chicken
2 large onions, finely chopped
4 garlic cloves, crushed
2 cinnamon sticks, broken in half
500 g (1 lb) sweet potatoes, cut into small cubes
500 g (1 lb) squash or pumpkin, cut into small cubes
small handful of chopped mixed parsley and mint
300 ml (½ pint) chicken stock
salt and pepper

To Garnish:
flaked almonds
parsley sprigs
mint sprigs

1 Heat the oil in a large heavy casserole. Add the chicken in batches and brown evenly. Remove and keep warm. Add the onions to the casserole and cook until soft and lightly browned, adding the garlic and cinnamon when the onions are nearly done.

2 Stir in the sweet potatoes and squash or pumpkin, then return the chicken to the pan, add half of the parsley and mint and pour in the stock. Cover tightly and simmer very gently for about 45 minutes until the chicken and vegetables are tender.

3 Season to taste with salt and pepper, then add the remaining parsley and mint. Scatter over the almonds and serve garnished with parsley and mint sprigs.

Pork, beef and lamb

Sweet and spicy pork with pomegranate

alcohol free ✕ | citrus free ✓ | dairy free ✓ | gluten free ✕ | wheat free ✕

Serves 2
Preparation time: 30 minutes
Cooking time: about 15 minutes

Per serving
Energy 553 kcals/2315 kJ | Protein 44 g | Carbohydrate 40 g | Fat 25 g
Saturated fat 7 g | Fibre 7 g

1 pork fillet (tenderloin), weighing about 375 g (12 oz)
2 tablespoons groundnut oil
4–7 spring onions, roughly chopped
2.5 cm (1 inch) piece of root ginger, finely chopped
2 garlic cloves, finely chopped
2–3 carrots, very thinly sliced diagonally
125 g (4 oz) bean sprouts
seeds of 1 pomegranate
salt and pepper

Sauce:
4 tablespoons Chinese rice wine or dry sherry
2 tablespoons soy sauce, or more to taste
2 tablespoons chilli sauce, or more to taste
2 tablespoons clear honey
1 tablespoon tomato purée
2 teaspoons cornflour

1 Cut the pork fillet crossways into 2 cm (¾ inch) slices, then cut these slices crossways into 2–3 strips. Mix the sauce ingredients in a measuring jug, add cold water up to the 250 ml (8 fl oz) mark and stir well to mix.

2 Heat an empty wok until hot. Add the oil and heat until very hot. Add the spring onions, ginger and garlic and stir-fry over a moderate heat for 1 minute. Add the carrots and stir-fry for 1–2 minutes.

3 Increase the heat to high, add the pork and stir-fry for 5 minutes. Pour in the sauce mixture and bring to the boil, stirring constantly, then simmer for about 2 minutes, or until the sauce is thick and reduced. Taste for seasoning and add more soy sauce or chilli sauce if liked.

4 Add the bean sprouts and toss vigorously to mix all the ingredients together, sprinkle with the pomegranate seeds and serve immediately.

Stir-fried pork
with tofu and mangetout

alcohol free ✗ | citrus free ✓ | dairy free ✓ | gluten free ✗ | wheat free ✗

Serves 3
Preparation time: 15–20 minutes
Cooking time: about 15 minutes

Per serving
Energy 416 kcals/1734 kJ | Protein 39 g | Carbohydrate 11 g | Fat 25 g
Saturated fat 6 g | Fibre 2 g

3 tablespoons groundnut oil
375 g (12 oz) pork fillet (tenderloin), cut into thin strips against
   the grain
250–300 g (8–10 oz) firm tofu, drained, dried and cut into cubes
125 g (4 oz) mangetout, trimmed
2 garlic cloves, crushed
250 g (8 oz) Chinese cabbage, shredded
pepper
1 teaspoon sesame oil, to finish

Sauce:
2 teaspoons cornflour
6 tablespoons chicken stock or water
3 tablespoons soy sauce
2 tablespoons Chinese rice wine or dry sherry
½ teaspoon Chinese five-spice powder
½ teaspoon chilli powder, or to taste

1 First prepare the sauce. Blend the cornflour to a paste with 2 tablespoons of the stock or water, then stir in the remaining stock or water and the rest of the sauce ingredients.

2 Heat an empty wok until hot. Add 2 tablespoons of the groundnut oil and heat until hot. Add the pork strips and stir-fry over a high heat for 3–4 minutes or until lightly coloured on all sides. Remove the wok from the heat and tip the pork and its juices into a bowl.

3 Return the wok to a moderate heat. Add the remaining groundnut oil and heat until hot. Add the tofu and stir-fry for 1–2 minutes or until lightly coloured on all sides. Remove the wok from the heat and transfer the tofu to kitchen paper with a slotted spoon. Keep hot.

4 Return the wok to the heat and add the mangetout and garlic. Stir-fry for 2 minutes. Return the pork and its juices to the wok, add the Chinese cabbage and stir-fry for 30 seconds, just until mixed with the pork and mangetout.

5 Stir the sauce to mix, then pour it into the wok. Increase the heat to high and stir for 1–2 minutes or until the sauce thickens. Gently fold in the tofu. Add pepper to taste and sprinkle with the sesame oil. Serve immediately.

Sweet and sour pork

alcohol free ✗ | citrus free ✓ | dairy free ✓ | gluten free ✗ | wheat free ✗

Serves 3
Preparation time: 15 minutes
Cooking time: 15 minutes

Per serving
Energy 519 kcals/2178 kJ | Protein 22 g | Carbohydrate 54 g | Fat 24 g
Saturated fat 4 g | Fibre 2 g

250 g (8 oz) pork, cut into cubes
1 teaspoon salt
1½ tablespoons brandy
1 egg, beaten
1 tablespoon cornflour
vegetable oil for deep-frying
125 g (4 oz) bamboo shoots, cut into chunks
1 green pepper, cored, deseeded and cut into chunks
2 spring onions, cut into 2.5 cm (1 inch) lengths
425 g (14 oz) can pineapple chunks in juice, drained and juice
    reserved

Sauce:
3 tablespoons vinegar
3 tablespoons sugar
½ teaspoon salt
1 tablespoon tomato purée
1 tablespoon soy sauce
1 tablespoon cornflour
1 teaspoon sesame oil

1 Place the pork in a bowl and sprinkle with the salt and brandy. Marinate in the refrigerator for 15 minutes. Add the beaten egg and cornflour and blend well.

2 Heat the oil in a wok to 180–190°C (350–375°F). Remove the wok from the heat but leave the pork in the oil for a further 2 minutes, then remove with a slotted spoon and drain on kitchen paper. Return the wok to the heat and reheat the pork with the bamboo shoots for 2 minutes. Remove and drain on kitchen paper.

3 Pour off the excess oil, leaving 1 tablespoonful in the wok. Add the green pepper and spring onions. Mix all the sauce ingredients with a little canned pineapple juice and add to the wok, stirring until thickened. Add the pork, bamboo shoots and pineapple chunks and serve hot.

Pork and vegetables

alcohol free ✕ ┃ citrus free ✓ ┃ dairy free ✓ ┃ gluten free ✕ ┃ wheat free ✕

Serves 3
Preparation time: 15 minutes
Cooking time: 8–10 minutes

Per serving
Energy 397 kcals/1653 kJ ┃ Protein 22 g ┃ Carbohydrate 20 g ┃ Fat 25 g
Saturated fat 4 g ┃ Fibre 6 g

2 tablespoons soy sauce

1 tablespoon dry sherry

2 teaspoons cornflour

250 g (8 oz) pork fillet, thinly sliced

5 tablespoons vegetable oil

2 spring onions, cut into 2.5 cm (1 inch) lengths

1 slice root ginger, finely chopped

125 g (4 oz) fresh bean sprouts

1 small green pepper, cored, deseeded and sliced

a few cauliflower or broccoli florets

2–3 tomatoes, cut into pieces

2 carrots, cut into pieces

50 g (2 oz) green beans, trimmed

2 teaspoons salt

1 tablespoon sugar

3 tablespoons chicken stock or water

rice, to serve

1 Mix together the soy sauce, sherry and cornflour in a bowl, and add the pork. Stir well until each slice is coated with the mixture.

2 Heat half of the oil in a wok. Add the sliced pork and stir-fry for 1 minute, then remove with a slotted spoon and set aside.

3 Heat the remaining oil and add the spring onions and ginger, followed by the bean sprouts, green pepper, cauliflower or broccoli, tomatoes, carrots, green beans, salt and sugar. Stir-fry for 1–2 minutes and then add the sliced pork. Moisten with a little stock or water if prefered and stir-fry quickly until the vegetables are tender but still crisp. Serve immediately with rice.

Beef with broccoli and oyster sauce

alcohol free ✗ | citrus free ✓ | dairy free ✓ | gluten free ✗ | wheat free ✗

Serves 2
Preparation time: about 15 minutes, plus freezing and marinating
Cooking time: 15–20 minutes

Per serving
Energy 486 kcals/2040 kJ | Protein 52 g | Carbohydrate 26 g | Fat 20 g
Saturated fat 6 g | Fibre 3 g

1 piece of rump steak, weighing about 375 g (12 oz), trimmed
   of all fat
1 egg white
2 tablespoons soy sauce
2 garlic cloves, crushed
2.5 cm (1 inch) piece of root ginger, grated
1 tablespoon cornflour
1 teaspoon sugar
about 50 ml (2 fl oz) groundnut oil, for frying
250 g (8 oz) broccoli, divided into small florets
125 ml (4 fl oz) Chinese rice wine or dry sherry
3 tablespoons oyster sauce
2 tablespoons soy sauce, or more to taste
salt and pepper

To Garnish:
sesame oil
2 tablespoons toasted sesame seeds
small bunch of chives, snipped (optional)

1 Wrap the beef in clingfilm and put it in the freezer for 1–2 hours until it is just hard.

2 Remove the beef from the freezer and unwrap it, then slice it into rectangles about the size of a large postage stamp, working against the grain. Whisk the egg white in a non-metallic dish, add the soy sauce, garlic, ginger, cornflour and sugar and whisk to mix. Add the beef, stir to coat, then leave to marinate at room temperature for about 30 minutes or until the beef is completely thawed out.

3 Heat the oil in a wok until very hot, but not smoking. Add about one-third of the beef rectangles and stir them around so they separate. Fry for 30–60 seconds until the beef changes colour all over, lift out with a slotted spoon and drain on kitchen paper. Repeat with the remaining beef. Very carefully pour off all but about 2 tablespoons of the hot oil from the wok.

4 Add the broccoli florets to the wok, sprinkle with the rice wine or sherry and toss over a moderate heat for 3 minutes. Return the beef to the wok and add the oyster sauce and soy sauce. Increase the heat to high and stir-fry vigorously for 3–4 minutes or until the beef and broccoli are tender. Taste for seasoning, and add more soy sauce if liked. Serve hot, drizzled with a little sesame oil and sprinkled with toasted sesame seeds. Garnish with snipped chives, if liked.

Chinese minced beef with tofu

alcohol free ✓ | citrus free ✓ | dairy free ✓ | gluten free ✓ | wheat free ✓

Serves 2
Preparation time: 10 minutes
Cooking time: about 10 minutes

Per serving
Energy 404 kcals/1685 kJ | Protein 28 g | Carbohydrate 16 g | Fat 26 g
Saturated fat 5 g | Fibre 1 g

2 teaspoons cornflour
150 ml (¼ pint) cold water
2 tablespoons soy sauce
2 tablespoons hoisin sauce
2 teaspoons chilli sauce
1 teaspoon dark soft brown sugar
2 tablespoons groundnut oil
125 g (4 oz) minced beef
2 teaspoons black bean sauce
6 button mushrooms, quartered lengthways
4 spring onions, thinly sliced into rings
3 garlic cloves, crushed
300 g (10 oz) tofu, drained, dried and diced
1 tablespoon sesame oil

To Serve:
½–1 teaspoon chilli oil, to taste
rice noodles (optional)

1 Blend the cornflour in a jug with 50 ml (2 fl oz) of the cold water, then add the remaining cold water, the soy, hoisin and chilli sauces and the sugar. Stir well to combine.

2 Heat an empty wok until hot. Add the oil and heat. Add the meat and black bean sauce, the mushrooms and half of the spring onions. Stir-fry over a high heat for 3–4 minutes. Add the garlic, the cornflour mixture and tofu and bring to the boil, stirring until thickened and glossy. Stir-fry for a further 2 minutes, then sprinkle with the remaining spring onions and the sesame oil. Serve drizzled with chilli oil to taste, accompanied by rice noodles if liked.

Paper-thin lamb
with garlic and spring onions

alcohol free ✗ | citrus free ✓ | dairy free ✓ | gluten free ✗ | wheat free ✗

Serves 3
Preparation time: 10 minutes, plus freezing
Cooking time: about 6 minutes

Per serving
Energy 364 kcals/1519 kJ | Protein 35 g | Carbohydrate 3 g | Fat 24 g
Saturated fat 8 g | Fibre 1 g

500 g (1 lb) lamb neck fillet, trimmed of fat and sinew
2 tablespoons groundnut oil
3 large garlic cloves, thinly sliced
½ teaspoon chilli powder, or to taste
½ teaspoon dark soft brown sugar
pinch of salt
1 large bunch of spring onions, cut into 7 cm (3 inch) lengths and
    shredded lengthways
2 tablespoons soy sauce
2 tablespoons Chinese rice wine or dry sherry
2 teaspoons sesame oil

1 Wrap the lamb in clingfilm and put it in the freezer for 1–2 hours until just hard. Cut it into paper-thin slices against the grain. Leave at room temperature for about 30 minutes or until completely thawed out.

2 Add the groundnut oil to a hot wok and heat. Add the garlic and stir-fry over a low heat for a few seconds to flavour the oil, then add the lamb and sprinkle with the chilli powder, sugar and salt. Increase the heat to high and stir-fry for 3–4 minutes until the lamb is browned.

3 Add the spring onions, soy sauce and rice wine or sherry and stir-fry for 30–60 seconds or until all the ingredients are quite dry. Serve immediately, sprinkled with the sesame oil.

Moroccan lamb

alcohol free ✓ | citrus free ✗ | dairy free ✓ | gluten free ✓ | wheat free ✓

Serves 4
Preparation time: 15 minutes, plus soaking
Cooking time: about 2½ hours

Per serving
Energy 622 kcals/2615 kJ | Protein 45 g | Carbohydrate 52 g | Fat 28 g
Saturated fat 7 g | Fibre 12 g

250 g (8 oz) chickpeas, soaked overnight
75 g (3 oz) dried apricots, soaked overnight
2 tablespoons vegetable oil
500 g (1 lb) lean, boneless lamb, cut into 1 cm (½ inch) cubes
1 large onion, chopped
1 garlic clove, crushed
300 ml (½ pint) chicken stock
2 tablespoons clear honey
1 teaspoon ground cinnamon
½ teaspoon ground allspice
½ teaspoon cumin seeds
very finely pared rind of ½ orange
salt and pepper

To Garnish:
50 g (2 oz) halved almonds, fried or toasted
1 tablespoon sesame seeds, toasted
mint sprigs

1 Drain the chickpeas. Drain the soaked apricots and cut them into small pieces. Heat 1 tablespoon of the oil in a flameproof casserole and fry the lamb until lightly browned and sealed all over. Remove from the casserole with a slotted spoon and set aside.

2 Add the remaining oil, onion and garlic to the casserole and fry very gently for about 5 minutes until soft. Add the stock and stir thoroughly.

3 Return the meat to the casserole and stir in the drained chickpeas. Cover closely with a lid or foil and cook on the centre shelf of a preheated oven, 160°C (325°F), Gas Mark 3, for 1 hour.

4 Add the honey, cinnamon, allspice, cumin seeds, orange rind and apricots and stir well together. Cover the casserole and return it to the oven for a further 1–1½ hours, or until the lamb is tender. Discard the orange rind.

5 Transfer the lamb to warm plates. Scatter the almonds over the top, sprinkle with sesame seeds and top with mint sprigs.

Vegetables and salads

Pesto chicken and pepper salad

alcohol free ✓ | citrus free ✓ | dairy free ✗ | gluten free ✓ | wheat free ✓

Serves 4
Preparation time: 20 minutes
Cooking time: 20 minutes

Per serving
Energy 329 kcals/1372 kJ | Protein 33 g | Carbohydrate 3 g | Fat 21 g
Saturated fat 5 g | Fibre 2 g

1 small cooked chicken
1 red pepper
1 yellow pepper
75 g (3 oz) mixed salad leaves (such as rocket, frisée, young spinach)
50 g (2 oz) black olives, pitted
olive oil, to drizzle
salt and pepper
basil sprigs, to garnish

Pesto Dressing:
15 g (½ oz) basil leaves
15 g (½ oz) Parmesan cheese, grated
2 tablespoons white wine vinegar
½ tablespoon pine nuts
1 small garlic clove, crushed
50 ml (2 fl oz) extra virgin olive oil

1 Skin the chicken and remove all the meat from the carcass. Shred the meat and set aside.

2 Cook the peppers under a preheated hot grill for 15–20 minutes, turning occasionally, until the skin is blackened all over. Transfer the peppers to a plastic bag and set aside to cool.

3 To make the pesto dressing, put the basil, Parmesan, vinegar, pine nuts and garlic into a food processor or blender, add pepper to taste and purée for a few seconds. With the motor running, drizzle the olive oil through the feeder tube until the mixture becomes thick and smooth.

4 When the peppers are cool enough to handle, rub off and discard the charred skin. Slice the flesh into thin strips, and discard the seeds and core. Season with salt and pepper.

5 Arrange the salad leaves in bowls. Pile the peppers on to the salad leaves, with the olives and chicken. Spoon the pesto over the chicken mixture. Serve immediately, drizzled with olive oil and garnished with basil sprigs.

Japanese seaweed salad

alcohol free ✗ | citrus free ✗ | dairy free ✓ | gluten free ✓ | wheat free ✓

Serves 4
Preparation time: 5–10 minutes, plus softening
Cooking time: 5 minutes

Per serving
Energy 50 kcals/215 kJ | Protein 4 g | Carbohydrate 10 g | Fat 0 g
Saturated fat 0 g | Fibre 3 g

25 g (1 oz) mixed dried seaweed, such as dulse or sea lettuce
wedges of lime or lemon, to serve

Mirin Dressing:
75 ml (3 fl oz) mirin (sweet Japanese rice wine)
75 ml (3 fl oz) rice wine vinegar
75 ml (3 fl oz) dashi (see page 115)
2 tablespoons caster sugar

1 Place the seaweed in a bowl, cover with cold water and leave for
15 minutes to soften.

2 To make the dressing, mix the mirin, vinegar and dashi in a small
saucepan with the sugar and heat gently until the sugar has
dissolved. Remove from the heat and leave to cool.

3 When the seaweed is soft, drain it well and arrange it on
individual plates. Dress with the mirin dressing. Serve with
wedges of lime or lemon to squeeze over the seaweed.

Roasted beetroot citrus salad

alcohol free ✓ | citrus free ✗ | dairy free ✓ | gluten free ✓ | wheat free ✓

Serves 6
Preparation time: 20 minutes
Cooking time: 35 minutes

Per serving
Energy 117 kcals/484 kJ | Protein 2 g | Carbohydrate 12 g | Fat: 7 g
Saturated fat 1 g | Fibre 2 g

6 beetroots, peeled and halved
4 Spanish onions, halved
50 ml (2 fl oz) olive oil
75 ml (3 fl oz) balsamic vinegar

Dressing:
1 tablespoon finely grated orange rind
50 ml (2 fl oz) fresh orange juice
50 ml (2 fl oz) olive oil
50 ml (2 fl oz) balsamic vinegar

1 Arrange the halved beetroots and onions in a single layer in an ovenproof dish. Mix together the oil and vinegar and pour it over the beetroots and onions. Bake in a preheated oven, 200°C (400°F), Gas Mark 6, for 35 minutes or until the beetroots are just tender. Transfer the beetroots and onions to a serving dish.

2 To make the dressing, place the orange rind in a bowl with the orange juice, oil and vinegar, and whisk to combine.

3 Pour the dressing over the beetroots and onions and serve immediately.

Three-bean fusilli salad

alcohol free ✓ | citrus free ✓ | dairy free ✗ | gluten free ✗ | wheat free ✗

Serves 4
Preparation time: 20 minutes
Cooking time: about 12 minutes

Per serving
Energy 420 kcals/1780 kJ | Protein 16 g | Carbohydrate 71 g | Fat 10 g
Saturated fat 6 g | Fibre 8 g

oil, see method
300 g (10 oz) dried tricolore fusilli
2 spring onions, chopped diagonally
1 red pepper, cored, deseeded and chopped
125 g (4 oz) drained canned red kidney beans
125 g (4 oz) drained canned pinto beans
125 g (4 oz) drained canned borlotti beans
200 ml (7 fl oz) half-fat crème fraĉche
4 tablespoons milk
3 tablespoons chopped dill
salt and pepper
dill sprigs, to garnish

1 Bring at least 1.8 litres (3 pints) water to the boil in a large
saucepan. Add a dash of oil and a generous pinch of salt. Cook
the pasta for 8–12 minutes, until just tender. Drain then rinse
under cold water in a colander, drain again and transfer to a
large salad bowl.

2 Add the spring onions, red pepper and beans. Mix well. Beat
together the crème fraĉche and milk in a bowl; fold into the salad
and add salt and pepper to taste. Fold in the chopped dill,
garnish with dill sprigs and serve.

Crispy seaweed

alcohol free ✓ | citrus free ✓ | dairy free ✓ | gluten free ✓ | wheat free ✓

Serves 8
Preparation time: 10 minutes, plus drying
Cooking time: 10 minutes

Per serving
Energy 70 kcals/293 kJ | Protein 3 g | Carbohydrate 4 g | Fat 5 g
Saturated fat 1 g | Fibre 6 g

750 g (1½ lb) spring greens, finely shredded
vegetable oil, for deep-frying
1½ teaspoons caster sugar
1 teaspoon salt

1 Spread out the shredded spring greens on kitchen paper for about 30 minutes until thoroughly dry.

2 Heat the oil in a wok to 180–190°C (350–375°F). Turn off the heat for 30 seconds and then add a small batch of shredded spring greens. Turn up the heat to moderate and deep-fry the greens until they begin to float on the surface of the oil. Take care, as they tend to spit while they are cooking.

3 Remove the greens with a slotted spoon and drain on kitchen paper. Cook the remaining greens in batches in the same way. When they are all cooked, transfer to a bowl and sprinkle over the sugar and salt. Toss gently to mix and serve warm or cold with Chinese dishes.

Sichuan tofu

alcohol free ✗ | citrus free ✓ | dairy free ✓ | gluten free ✓ | wheat free ✓

Serves 4
Preparation time: 15 minutes, plus soaking
Cooking time: about 15 minutes

Per serving
Energy 147 kcals/613 kJ | Protein 8 g | Carbohydrate 8 g | Fat 9 g
Saturated fat 2 g | Fibre 1 g

6 dried shiitake mushrooms
125 ml (4 fl oz) hot water
2 tablespoons groundnut oil
4 spring onions, cut crossways into quarters
1 small red pepper, cored, deseeded and finely diced
1 small green pepper, cored, deseeded and finely diced
2 garlic cloves, finely chopped
1 bird's eye chilli, deseeded and very finely chopped
2 heaped tablespoons canned salted black beans, rinsed and
  coarsely mashed
2 tablespoons black bean sauce
2 tablespoons Chinese rice wine or dry sherry
4 tablespoons cold water
300 g (10 oz) firm tofu, drained, dried and cut into 2.5–4 cm
  (1–1½ inch) squares
salt and pepper
chilli oil, to finish

1 Soak the dried mushrooms in the hot water for 35–40 minutes. Drain the mushrooms in a sieve over a bowl and reserve the soaking water. Cut the mushroom caps into small squares, discarding any hard stalks.

2 Heat an empty wok until hot. Add the oil and heat until hot. Add the spring onions, red and green peppers, garlic, chilli and mushrooms, stir-fry for 1–2 minutes, then add the black beans and black bean sauce, the rice wine or sherry, the mushroom soaking liquid and the cold water. Bring to the boil and simmer for 5 minutes, then add the tofu and stir gently to mix. Simmer for another 5 minutes, stirring occasionally. Taste for seasoning and serve hot, drizzled with chilli oil.

Green beans with broccoli and almonds

alcohol free ✓ | citrus free ✗ | dairy free ✓ | gluten free ✗ | wheat free ✗

Serves 4
Preparation time: 10–15 minutes
Cooking time: about 12 minutes

Per serving
Energy 170 kcals/707 kJ | Protein 6 g | Carbohydrate 7 g | Fat 13 g
Saturated fat 2 g | Fibre 3 g

2 teaspoons cornflour

6 tablespoons vegetable stock or water

2 tablespoons soy sauce

1 tablespoon lemon juice

4 tablespoons flaked almonds

2 tablespoons groundnut oil

175 g (6 oz) broccoli, separated into small florets

175 g (6 oz) green beans, cut diagonally into 4–5 cm (1½–2 inch lengths)

3 garlic cloves, crushed

pepper

1 Blend the cornflour in a jug with 2 tablespoons of the stock or water, then add the remaining stock or water and the soy sauce and lemon juice. Stir well to combine.

2 Dry-fry the flaked almonds in a wok over a moderate heat for 1–2 minutes until they are lightly toasted, then remove them and set aside.

3 Heat the oil in the wok until hot, add the broccoli and stir-fry for 3 minutes. Add the beans and garlic and stir-fry for 3–4 minutes.

4 Pour in the cornflour mixture and bring to the boil over a high heat, stirring constantly until thickened. Add pepper to taste and serve sprinkled with the almonds.

Steamed vegetables with ginger

alcohol free ✓ | citrus free ✓ | dairy free ✓ | gluten free ✓ | wheat free ✓

Serves 4
Preparation time: 10 minutes
Cooking time: 7 minutes

Per serving
Energy 54 kcals/226 kJ | Protein 3 g | Carbohydrate 9 g | Fat 1 g
Saturated fat 0 g | Fibre 2 g

3 carrots, cut into 5 mm (¼ inch) rounds
75 g (3 oz) cauliflower florets
75 g (3 oz) broccoli florets
2 small courgettes, cut into 1 cm (½ inch) rounds
3.5 cm (1½ inch) piece root ginger, cut into thin strips

1 Place all the vegetables in a steamer with the ginger and steam
over boiling water for 7 minutes until tender.

Stir-fried mixed vegetables

alcohol free ✓ | citrus free ✓ | dairy free ✓ | gluten free ✓ | wheat free ✓

Serves 4
Preparation time: 15 minutes
Cooking time: 6–7 minutes

Per serving
Energy 137 kcals/569 kJ | Protein 5 g | Carbohydrate 9 g | Fat 10 g
Saturated fat 1 g | Fibre 4 g

3 tablespoons vegetable oil
1 garlic clove, crushed
125 g (4 oz) cabbage, shredded
125 g (4 oz) cauliflower, divided into florets
125 g (4 oz) broccoli, divided into florets
½ teaspoon pepper
2 tablespoons oyster sauce
150 ml (¼ pint) chicken or vegetable stock
2 carrots, cut into matchstick strips
125 g (4 oz) mushrooms, thinly sliced
1 onion, sliced
50 g (2 oz) bean sprouts

1 Heat the oil in a wok. Add the crushed garlic and stir-fry quickly over moderate heat until golden. Do not let it get too brown.

2 Add the shredded cabbage, cauliflower, broccoli, and the black pepper. Stir in the oyster sauce and the chicken or vegetable stock and then cook, stirring constantly, for 3 minutes.

3 Add the carrots, mushrooms and onion to the wok together with the bean sprouts. Stir-fry for 2 minutes. Transfer the fried vegetables to a large dish or platter and serve immediately.

Caponata

alcohol free ✓ | citrus free ✓ | dairy free ✓ | gluten free ✓ | wheat free ✓

Serves 6
Preparation time: 20 minutes, plus standing
Cooking time: about 1¼ hours

Per serving
Energy 83 kcals/347 kJ | Protein 3 g | Carbohydrate 5 g | Fat 6 g
Saturated fat 1 g | Fibre 3 g

3 aubergines, cut into 1 cm (½ inch) dice
2 tablespoons olive oil
1 onion, thinly sliced
2 celery sticks, diced
150 ml (¼ pint) passata (Italian chopped tomatoes)
3 tablespoons wine vinegar
1 yellow pepper, cored, deseeded and thinly sliced
1 red pepper, cored, deseeded and thinly sliced
25 g (1 oz) anchovy fillets, soaked in warm water, drained and dried
50 g (2 oz) capers, roughly chopped
25 g (1 oz) black olives, pitted and sliced
25 g (1 oz) green olives, pitted and sliced
salt
2 tablespoons chopped parsley, to serve

1 Put the diced aubergines into a colander, sprinkle with salt and leave to drain for 15–20 minutes to exude their bitter juices. Rinse under cold running water to remove any salt and pat dry with kitchen paper.

2 Heat the oil in a saucepan, add the onion and sauté until soft and golden. Add the celery and cook for 2–3 minutes. Add the aubergine and cook gently for 3 minutes, stirring occasionally. Add the passata and cook gently until it has been absorbed. Add the wine vinegar and cook for 1 minute. Add the peppers, anchovies, capers and olives and cook for 3 minutes.

3 Transfer the mixture to an ovenproof dish and bake, covered, in a preheated oven, 180°C (350°F), Gas Mark 4, for about 1 hour. Serve lukewarm or cold, sprinkled with chopped parsley.

Chinese braised vegetables

alcohol free ✓ | citrus free ✓ | dairy free ✓ | gluten free ✕ | wheat free ✕

Serves 4
Preparation time: 20 minutes
Cooking time: 15 minutes

Per serving
Energy 223 kcals/929 kJ | Protein 9 g | Carbohydrate 14 g | Fat 15 g
Saturated fat 2 g | Fibre 2 g

5–6 Chinese dried mushrooms, soaked in warm water for 20 minutes
250 g (8 oz) firm tofu, cut into cubes
4 tablespoons vegetable oil
125 g (4 oz) carrots, sliced
125 g (4 oz) mangetout, trimmed
125 g (4 oz) Chinese leaves, shredded
2 spring onions, cut into 1 cm (½ inch) lengths
125 g (4 oz) bamboo shoots, sliced
1 teaspoon sugar
1 tablespoon light soy sauce
1 teaspoon cornflour
1 tablespoon cold water
1 teaspoon sesame oil
salt

1 Drain the dried mushrooms and squeeze them dry. Discard the hard stalks and cut the caps into thin slices.

2 Bring a saucepan of lightly salted water to the boil and add the tofu. Boil for 2–3 minutes until firm. Remove the tofu pieces with a slotted spoon and drain well on kitchen paper.

3 Heat about half of the oil in a wok. Add the tofu and fry until lightly browned. Remove with a slotted spoon and set aside.

4 Heat the remaining oil in the wok. Add the vegetables and stir-fry for 2 minutes. Stir in the tofu with 1 teaspoon salt, the sugar and soy sauce. Cover, reduce the heat and braise for 3 minutes.

5 Meanwhile, mix the cornflour to a smooth paste with the water. Stir into the braised vegetables in the wok. Increase the heat and continue stirring until the sauce thickens. Sprinkle in the sesame oil and serve immediately.

Pasta, rice and noodles

Broccoli and red pepper fettuccine salad

alcohol free ✓ | citrus free ✓ | dairy free ✓ | gluten free ✕ | wheat free ✕

Serves 4
Preparation time: 10 minutes
Cooking time: about 15 minutes

Per serving
Energy 375 kcals/1510 kJ | Protein 13 g | Carbohydrate 51 g | Fat 14 g
Saturated fat 2 g | Fibre 1 g

4 tablespoons olive oil
300 g (10 oz) fresh fettuccine
3 red peppers, cored, deseeded and halved
250 g (8 oz) small broccoli florets
2 tablespoons balsamic vinegar
salt and pepper
basil leaves, to garnish

1 Bring at least 1.8 litres (3 pints) water to the boil in a large saucepan. Add a dash of oil and a pinch of salt. Cook the pasta for 4–6 minutes, until just tender. Drain, rinse under cold running water in a colander and drain again. Set aside in a large salad bowl.

2 Grill the peppers, skin side up, until the skins have blackened and blistered. Remove from the heat and leave to cool for 5 minutes.

3 Meanwhile, bring a large saucepan of lightly salted water to the boil and blanch the broccoli florets for 3 minutes. Drain, rinse under cold running water and drain again.

4 Peel the peppers and slice the flesh into strips. Add to the pasta with the drained broccoli florets, the remaining olive oil and the balsamic vinegar. Add salt and pepper to taste and toss well. Serve immediately, garnished with basil leaves.

Tagliatelle with chilli and roast cherry tomato dressing

alcohol free ✓ | citrus free ✕ | dairy free ✓ | gluten free ✕ | wheat free ✕

Serves 4
Preparation time: 10 minutes
Cooking time: 15 minutes

Per serving
Energy 574 kcals/2305 kJ | Protein 18 g | Carbohydrate 79 g | Fat 21 g
Saturated fat 3 g | Fibre 2 g

250 g (8 oz) cherry tomatoes
2 teaspoons ready-made pesto
4 tablespoons olive oil, plus a dash
2 spring onions, thinly sliced
1 red or green chilli, deseeded and finely chopped
2 garlic cloves, chopped
1 tablespoon raspberry vinegar
1 tablespoon orange juice
2 tablespoons toasted hazelnuts, chopped
2 tablespoons chopped basil
500 g (1 lb) fresh tagliatelle verde
salt and pepper
a few basil leaves, to garnish

1 Halve the tomatoes and arrange them on a baking sheet. Sprinkle with a little salt and top with pesto. Toss carefully, making sure you coat the tomatoes well. Cook in a preheated oven, 200°C (400°F), Gas Mark 6, for 15 minutes.

2 Meanwhile, heat the olive oil in a small saucepan. Add the spring onions, chilli and garlic and fry for 1 minute, stirring continuously. Remove from the heat, add the vinegar, orange juice, hazelnuts and basil. Stir well, season and keep warm.

3 Meanwhile, bring at least 1.8 litres (3 pints) water to the boil in a large saucepan. Add a dash of oil and a generous pinch of salt. Just before the tomatoes are ready, cook the pasta for 4 minutes or according to the packet instructions. Drain the pasta and return it to the pan. Add the spring onion mixture and toss well. Add the tomatoes and all the cooking juices. Serve garnished with basil.

Spaghetti with marinated vegetables

alcohol free ✓ | citrus free ✓ | dairy free ✓ | gluten free ✕ | wheat free ✕

Serves 4
Preparation time: 20 minutes, plus chilling
Cooking time: 25 minutes

Per serving
Energy 480 kcals/2015 kJ | Protein 11 g | Carbohydrate 59 g | Fat 24 g
Saturated fat 3 g | Fibre 7 g

1 red pepper, halved, cored and deseeded
1 tablespoon salt
1 small aubergine, sliced
125 g (4 oz) flat field mushrooms
1 leek, trimmed, cleaned and thinly sliced
1 teaspoon cumin seeds
½ teaspoon coriander seeds
150 ml (¼ pint) raspberry vinegar
8 tablespoons olive oil
1 tablespoon garlic purée
300 g (10 oz) dried spaghetti
salt and pepper

To Garnish:
mixed salad leaves
flat leaf parsley

1 Place the red pepper halves on a grill pan, skin side up, and grill under a high heat for about 10 minutes until the skin is blackened and blistered. Remove from the heat and leave them to cool.

2 Meanwhile, sprinkle the salt over the aubergine slices and set aside for 15 minutes. Drain the aubergine slices, rinse them well and pat dry with kitchen paper. Place on a grill pan, and grill under a high heat for 10 minutes, turning the slices once, until browned. Remove from the grill pan and set aside. Add the mushrooms to the grill pan and grill for 2 minutes.

3 Peel the pepper and finely slice the flesh. Slice the mushrooms. Combine all the grilled vegetables in a large bowl and add the leek. Stir in the spices, vinegar, oil and garlic purée with salt and pepper to taste. Toss the mixture until combined, and set aside.

4 Bring at least 1.8 litres (3 pints) water to the boil in a large saucepan. Add a dash of oil and a generous pinch of salt. Cook the pasta for 8–12 minutes, until just tender. Drain thoroughly and add to the vegetable mixture. Toss again and chill for 3 hours before serving.

5 Serve garnished with salad leaves and flat leaf parsley.

Pasta niçoise

alcohol free ✓ | citrus free ✓ | dairy free ✓ | gluten free ✕ | wheat free ✕

Serves 4
Preparation time: 20 minutes, plus chilling
Cooking time: 12 minutes

Per serving
Energy 405 kcals/1700 kJ | Protein 12 g | Carbohydrate 60 g | Fat 15 g
Saturated fat 2 g | Fibre 6 g

300 g (10 oz) dried fusilli
250 g (8 oz) green beans, trimmed, halved and cooked
25 g (1 oz) anchovy fillets
2 teaspoons capers, chopped
25 g (1 oz) pitted black olives
1 large ripe plum tomato, cut lengthways into eighths
salt and pepper
1 tablespoon basil leaves, to garnish

Dressing:
4 tablespoons olive oil
2 tablespoons sherry vinegar
1 teaspoon Dijon mustard
pinch of sugar

1 Bring at least 1.8 litres (3 pints) water to the boil in a large saucepan. Add a dash of oil and a generous pinch of salt. Cook the fusilli for 8–12 minutes, until just tender. Drain the pasta and rinse under cold running water in a colander. Drain again and set aside while preparing the salad.

2 Place the French beans in a bowl with the anchovy fillets, capers, olives and tomato. Add plenty of salt and pepper to taste. Add the pasta and toss well.

3 Make the dressing. Place the oil, vinegar, mustard and sugar in a screw-top jar. Close the jar tightly and shake well. Pour over the salad, toss again and sprinkle with the basil leaves. Chill in the refrigerator until required.

Spaghetti marinara

alcohol free ✕ | citrus free ✓ | dairy free ✕ | gluten free ✕ | wheat free ✕

Serves 4
Preparation time: 20 minutes
Cooking time: 12 minutes

Per serving
Energy 440 kcals/1860 kJ | Protein 23 g | Carbohydrate 61 g | Fat 11 g
Saturated fat 4 g | Fibre 4 g

oil, see method
300 g (10 oz) dried spaghetti
25 g (1 oz) butter
25 g (1 oz) plain flour
125 ml (4 fl oz) dry white wine
125 ml (4 fl oz) hot vegetable stock
125 g (4 oz) squid, cut into rings
125 g (4 oz) salmon steak, boned and cubed
50 g (2 oz) cooked peeled prawns
salt and pepper
1 tablespoon chopped fennel fronds, to garnish

1 Bring at least 1.8 litres (3 pints) water to the boil in a large
saucepan. Add a dash of oil and a generous pinch of salt. Cook
the pasta for 8–12 minutes, until just tender.

2 Meanwhile, melt the butter in a saucepan, stir in the flour and
cook for about 1 minute. Gradually add the wine and the stock,
whisking or beating the sauce over a moderate heat until
thickened. Add salt and pepper to taste, stir in the squid, salmon
and prawns and then simmer for 5 minutes.

3 Drain the pasta and return it to the rinsed saucepan. Add the fish
sauce and toss lightly. Serve garnished with the fennel fronds.

Spaghetti with anchovies and olives

alcohol free ✓ | citrus free ✓ | dairy free ✕ | gluten free ✕ | wheat free ✕

Serves 4
Preparation time: 10 minutes
Cooking time: 12–14 minutes

Per serving
Energy 407 kcals/1720 kJ | Protein 13 g | Carbohydrate 70 g | Fat 10 g
Saturated fat 4 g | Fibre 5 g

oil, see method
375 g (12 oz) dried spaghetti
25 g (1 oz) butter
6 drained canned anchovy fillets, chopped
1 tablespoon tomato purée
1 tablespoon olive paste
6 pitted black olives, chopped
salt and pepper
bunch of fresh basil
Parmesan shavings, to garnish

1 Bring at least 1.8 litres (3 pints) water to the boil in a large saucepan. Add a dash of oil and a generous pinch of salt. Cook the pasta for 8–12 minutes, until just tender.

2 Drain the pasta and set it aside. Melt the butter in a large saucepan. Add the anchovy fillets, tomato purée, olive paste and olives. Stir over the heat until the mixture sizzles. Season well with pepper. Cool for 1 minute.

3 Add the drained pasta to the saucepan. Toss well. Tear the basil leaves and add them to the pasta. Serve with Parmesan shavings.

Seafood risotto

alcohol free ✓ | citrus free ✓ | dairy free ✕ | gluten free ✓ | wheat free ✓

Serves 4
Preparation time: 10 minutes
Cooking time: about 25 minutes

Per serving
Energy 489 kcals/2064 kJ | Protein 32 g | Carbohydrate 64 g | Fat 13 g
Saturated fat 8 g | Fibre 4 g

50 g (2 oz) butter
1 onion, chopped
1 yellow pepper, cored, deseeded and chopped
1 red pepper, cored, deseeded and chopped
4 tomatoes, skinned, deseeded and chopped
375 g (12 oz) cod, skinned and cut into bite-sized pieces
8 scallops, cleaned
250 g (8 oz) Italian risotto rice
475 ml (16 fl oz) hot fish stock
salt and pepper
1 tablespoon finely chopped parsley, to garnish
2 tablespoons grated Parmesan cheese, to serve

1 Melt half of the butter in a saucepan, add the onion, yellow and red peppers and tomatoes and fry gently for 1 minute, stirring occasionally.

2 Add the cod and scallops, and fry for a further 3 minutes. Transfer to a bowl and season to taste with salt and pepper. Cover and set aside.

3 Melt the remaining butter in the pan, add the rice and fry for 3 minutes, stirring. Stir in the stock and 1 teaspoon of salt. Bring to the boil, lower the heat and cover the pan. Simmer for 15 minutes until the rice is almost tender and the liquid has been absorbed. Gently stir in the cod mixture and heat for 2 minutes.

4 Garnish the risotto with parsley, sprinkle with the Parmesan cheese and serve immediately.

Fish risotto

alcohol free ✗ | citrus free ✓ | dairy free ✗ | gluten free ✓ | wheat free ✓

Serves 6
Preparation time: 20 minutes
Cooking time: 45–55 minutes

Per serving
Energy 494 kcals/2084 kJ | Protein 38 g | Carbohydrate 58 g | Fat 12 g
Saturated fat 6 g | Fibre 2 g

50 g (2 oz) unsalted butter
1 large onion, finely chopped
1.2–1.5 litres (2–2½ pints) fish stock
1 celery stick, sliced
1 thyme sprig
2 parsley sprigs
1 mace blade
1 small onion, studded with 2 cloves
375–500 g (12 oz–1 lb) Italian risotto rice
150 ml (¼ pint) dry white wine
500 g (1 lb) monkfish, haddock, halibut or other firm white fillets,
   skinned and cubed
2 small red mullet, heads and tails removed, cut into 2.5 mm
   (1 inch) slices (optional)
3–4 saffron threads (optional)
1 garlic clove, finely chopped
300 g (10 oz) cooked shelled prawns
40 g (1½ oz) grated Parmesan cheese, plus extra to serve
sea salt and white pepper
finely chopped parsley, to garnish

1 Heat 15 g (½ oz) of the butter in a large pan, add the onion and cook for 5–10 minutes until soft, but not coloured.

2 Meanwhile, put the fish stock into another pan, then tie the celery, thyme, parsley, mace blade and studded onion in a piece of muslin and add to the pan. Bring just to boiling point, then simmer.

3 Add the rice (use a larger amount if omitting the mullet) to the onion, and stir until well coated with butter. Pour in the wine and cook for 3–4 minutes until the wine has almost evaporated.

4 Add a ladleful, or about 125 ml (4 fl oz), of the hot stock to the pan and cook over a low heat for 2–4 minutes, until the stock is almost absorbed, then add another ladleful, stirring it into the rice. Continue adding the stock, a little at a time, and stirring frequently to prevent sticking, until you have added about 1 litre (1¾ pints). By this time, you should be stirring almost constantly. Add the monkfish and red mullet slices, if using, then a little more stock and cook for 4–5 minutes.

5 Put the saffron, if using, into a small bowl and pour over 3–4 tablespoons of the stock. Stir quickly to start the colour running, then set aside.

6 Melt 15 g (½ oz) of the remaining butter in another small pan, add the garlic and prawns and cook for 3–4 minutes, then stir into the risotto. Add the saffron liquid, and another ladleful of stock if you have used the whole quantity of the rice. The rice should be tender and the risotto creamy and moist without being 'gluey', so be careful at this stage – it is easy to make it too liquid. Season with salt and pepper.

7 Add the remaining butter and the Parmesan, stirring until melted, then pile into a warmed serving dish. Sprinkle with parsley and serve immediately with more Parmesan.

Malaysian chicken, noodle and prawn stew

alcohol free ✗ | citrus free ✓ | dairy free ✓ | gluten free ✗ | wheat free ✗

Serves 6
Preparation time: 20 minutes
Cooking time: 30 minutes

Per serving
Energy 373 kcals/1555 kJ | Protein 22 g | Carbohydrate 22 g | Fat 22 g
Saturated fat 14 g | Fibre 4 g

2 tablespoons oil
4–6 spring onions, shredded
5 cm (2 inch) piece of root ginger, cut into very thin matchsticks
2 garlic cloves, crushed
375 g (12 oz) boneless, skinless chicken breasts, cut diagonally into
   thin strips
2 tablespoons Chinese rice wine or dry sherry
2 tablespoons soy sauce
1 teaspoon ground turmeric
1 teaspoon chilli powder
1.8 litres (3 pints) chicken stock
2 tablespoons Thai fish sauce or light soy sauce
125 g (4 oz) creamed coconut, roughly chopped
2 carrots, cut into very thin matchsticks
250 g (8 oz) green beans, cut diagonally into 5 cm (2 inch) lengths
375 g (12 oz) Chinese egg noodles
125 g (4 oz) bean sprouts
8–12 large raw prawns in their shells
salt and pepper

1 Heat the oil in a large flameproof casserole and stir-fry the spring onions, ginger and garlic for about 5 minutes until softened, but not coloured. Add the chicken and stir-fry until it changes colour, then stir in the rice wine or sherry, soy sauce, turmeric, chilli powder and salt and pepper to taste.

2 Gradually add the stock and fish sauce, stirring constantly to mix with the chicken and flavouring ingredients. Add the creamed coconut and simmer, stirring occasionally, for about 5 minutes, until the coconut has dissolved. Cover and simmer gently for about 10 minutes until the chicken is just tender.

3 Add the carrots and green beans, cover and simmer for a further 5 minutes. Add the noodles, bean sprouts and prawns, cover and remove from the heat. Leave to stand for 5 minutes until the noodles are soft and the prawns pink.

4 Remove the prawns from the casserole and pull off their shells with your fingers. Slice the prawns horizontally in half, then return to the casserole and stir well to mix. Adjust the seasoning to taste and serve hot, in warmed bowls.

Desserts

Yogurt-fruit cup

alcohol free ✓ | citrus free ✓ | dairy free ✗ | gluten free ✓ | wheat free ✓

Serves 6
Preparation time: 10 minutes

Per serving
Energy 134 kcals/568 kJ | Protein 5 g | Carbohydrate 23 g | Fat 4 g
Saturated fat 1 g | Fibre 1 g

500 g (1 lb) can sliced peaches or pears in fruit juice, drained
475 ml (16 fl oz) low-fat vanilla yogurt
2 tablespoons finely chopped toasted almonds
½ teaspoon ground cardamom

1 Divide the fruit among 6 goblets or small dessert bowls. Top with yogurt and sprinkle lightly with the nuts and cardamom. Serve immediately.

Summer fruit platter

alcohol free ✗ | citrus free ✓ | dairy free ✓ | gluten free ✓ | wheat free ✓

Serves 4
Preparation time: 10 minutes, plus chilling

Per serving
Energy 107 kcals/453 kJ | Protein 2 g | Carbohydrate 21 g | Fat 0 g
Saturated fat 0 g | Fibre 7 g

175 g (6 oz) cherries
2 kiwifruit, peeled and sliced
1 peach, pitted and sliced
125 g (4 oz) redcurrant sprigs
125 g (4 oz) strawberries, sliced

Raspberry Sauce:
150 g (5 oz) raspberries
1 tablespoon clear honey
2 tablespoons Crème de Framboise liqueur

1 First make the sauce. Put the raspberries into a food processor or blender with the honey and blend until smooth. Work the purée through a sieve to remove the seeds, then stir in the liqueur. Cover and chill until ready to serve.

2 Pour a pool of sauce on one side of each serving plate and arrange the fruits attractively on the other side.

Strawberries with blackcurrant sauce

alcohol free ✗ | citrus free ✓ | dairy free ✓ | gluten free ✓ | wheat free ✓

Serves 4
Preparation time: 25 minutes, plus cooling
Cooking time: 5 minutes

Per serving
Energy 79 kcals/336 kJ | Protein 1 g | Carbohydrate 17 g | Fat 0 g
Saturated fat 0 g | Fibre 7 g

250 g (8 oz) blackcurrants, trimmed
2 tablespoons clear honey
3 tablespoons red wine
375 g (12 oz) strawberries, hulled and halved
small redcurrant sprigs, to decorate

1 Put the blackcurrants into a pan with the honey and red wine;
stir well, then simmer gently for about 5 minutes or until the
natural fruit juices are released.

2 Pour the blackcurrants and their liquid into a food processor or
blender and purée until fairly smooth, the sauce should still have
some texture. Leave to cool.

3 To serve, arrange the halved strawberries on a serving dish.
Spoon the blackcurrant sauce beside them and decorate with the
redcurrant sprigs.

Stuffed figs

alcohol free ✓ I citrus free ✓ I dairy free ✓ I gluten free ✓ I wheat free ✓

Serves 4
Preparation time: 10–15 minutes

Per serving
Energy 100 kcals/424 kJ I Protein 4 g I Carbohydrate 8 g I Fat 6 g
Saturated fat 1 g I Fibre 5 g

12 ripe fresh figs, preferably purple ones
3 tablespoons ground almonds
125 g (4 oz) fresh raspberries
1 tablespoon clear honey
4 vine leaves, soaked in warm water and dried, to serve

1 Snip off any excess stalk from each fig. Make a criss-cross cut down from the stalk end and carefully ease the cut open.

2 Mix the ground almonds with the fresh raspberries and honey.

3 Place a vine leaf, spread out flat, on each serving plate. Arrange three figs on top of each one and fill with the raspberry and almond purée.

Melon ice cream

alcohol free ✓ | citrus free ✓ | dairy free ✗ | gluten free ✓ | wheat free ✓

Serves 4
Preparation time: 20–25 minutes, plus freezing

Per serving
Energy 90 kcals/380 kJ | Protein 5 g | Carbohydrate 16 g | Fat 1 g
Saturated fat 0 g | Fibre 2 g

1 large melon (Ogen or Charentais)
300 ml (½ pint) natural yogurt

1 Halve the melon and scoop out all the seeds. Scoop the melon flesh into a food processor or blender and work until smooth.

2 Mix the melon purée with the yogurt. Transfer the melon and yogurt mixture to a shallow freezer container, and freeze until firm.

3 Serve the melon ice cream in scoops.

Spiced pears

alcohol free ✕ | citrus free ✕ | dairy free ✓ | gluten free ✓ | wheat free ✓

Serves 4
Preparation time: 20 minutes
Cooking time: about 16 minutes

Per serving
Energy 180 kcals/760 kJ | Protein 1 g | Carbohydrate 33 g | Fat 0 g
Saturated fat 0 g | Fibre 6 g

4 large firm pears
½ lemon
16 cloves
½ cinnamon stick
300 ml (½ pint) red wine
2 tablespoons redcurrant jelly
4 orange slices
4 small fresh bay leaves, to decorate

1 Peel the pears, leaving the stalks intact. Rub them all over with the lemon half to prevent discoloration. Stud each pear with 4 cloves. Stand them upright in a pan and add the cinnamon stick, wine and sufficient water just to cover the pears. Bring to the boil and simmer gently until the pears are just tender. Leave to cool in the cooking liquid.

2 Put 2 tablespoons of the cooking liquid into a small pan with the redcurrant jelly. Bubble briskly for about 1 minute until the jelly has dissolved.

3 Place an orange slice on each of 4 small plates. Lift out the pears with a slotted spoon, and sit one on top of each orange slice. Spoon a little of the redcurrant glaze over each pear and decorate with a bay leaf.

Melon, grape and kiwifruit salad

alcohol free ✗ | citrus free ✓ | dairy free ✓ | gluten free ✓ | wheat free ✓

Serves 4
Preparation time: 10 minutes, plus chilling

Per serving
Energy 165 kcals/704 kJ | Protein 2 g | Carbohydrate 38 g | Fat 0 g
Saturated fat 0 g | Fibre 2 g

1 large Galia melon
125 g (4 oz) seedless green grapes, skinned
3 kiwifruit, thinly sliced
325 g (11 oz) canned lychees, drained
2 apples, peeled, cored and thinly sliced
3 tablespoons kirsch
mint sprigs, to decorate

1 Cut a thin slice from the base of the melon so that it stands firm. Slice the top off the melon, remove the seeds and discard. Scoop out the flesh in small balls, using a melon baller or a teaspoon. Reserve the shell.

2 Place the melon balls in a bowl with the grapes, kiwifruit, lychees and apples and sprinkle with the kirsch. Cover and chill until ready to serve.

3 Place the melon shell on a serving plate. Pile the fruit into the shell and decorate with mint sprigs.

Glossary

ANTIOXIDANTS Vitamins (C, E and beta-carotene, which is converted into vitamin A in the body) that help to control the unstable molecules, called free radicals, that attack body cells.

CLIMACTERIC The complete process of hormonal changes from the time when oestrogen levels start to drop to a few years after the menopause.

FREE RADICALS Chemicals produced naturally in the body which limit the effectiveness of the immune system.

FSH Follicle-stimulating hormone, released by the pituitary gland in the brain. FSH causes one of the egg-containing follicles in the ovaries to mature.

HOLISTIC   An approach taken by many complementary therapies, that involves treating the whole person, not just the disease they happen to be suffering from.

HOT FLUSH   A burning sensation and reddening of the skin, usually felt across the face, neck and chest, caused by fluctuating hormone levels.

HRT   Hormone replacement therapy, that corrects the balance of hormones whose fluctuations cause menopausal symptoms.

HYPOTHALAMUS   A gland at the base of the brain that, among other things, controls the menstrual cycle by releasing hormones.

LH   Luteinizing hormone, secreted by the pituitary gland, which causes the ovary to release an egg.

LIBIDO   Sex drive.

MENOPAUSE   A woman's very last period, a diagnosis that can only be made after the event when it is clear no more periods will occur.

NUTRICEUTICALS   A term used by nutritionists to describe foods that have a positive therapeutic or medicinal effect on the body.

OESTROGEN   The hormone produced by the ovaries that helps to regulate the menstrual cycle and reproductive system.

OSTEOPOROSIS A weakening of the bones caused by a drop in oestrogen in the body. The bones become less dense and rather brittle as old bone is lost but new bone is not replaced as quickly as before.

PATCHES Thin sticky patches that are applied to the skin to release HRT hormones slowly into the body.

PERI-MENOPAUSE The period covering the few years either side of the menopause.

PHYTOESTROGENS Plant foods that produce natural oestrogens. When eaten, they can increase the level of oestrogen in the body.

PITUITARY GLAND A gland at the base of the brain that works with the hypothalamus to regulate the menstrual cycle.

PMS Premenstrual syndrome, the emotional and physical symptoms that occur in the week before a period.

POST-MENOPAUSE The period of a few years immediately after the final period.

PRE-MENOPAUSE The phase when hormone levels begin to change in the run-up to the menopause.

PROGESTERONE The female hormone that, with oestrogen, helps regulate the menstrual cycle and prepare the body for pregnancy.

PROGESTOGEN A synthetic form of progesterone, used in HRT.

REGIMEN A word used by doctors to describe a prescribed course of treatment.

SUBCUTANEOUS HRT Hormone replacement therapy in the form of a hormone-releasing implant that is effective for 3–6 months.

TESTOSTERONE The masculinizing hormone, also present in women, whose effects become more apparent as the female hormones decline.

TIBOLONE A synthetic, non-hormonal alternative to HRT that has many of the same health benefits but does not cause a regular 'period'.

TRANSDERMAL HRT Hormone replacement therapy applied to the skin in the form of hormone-releasing gels and patches.

UTERUS The womb.

General index

A

acupuncture 73, 78–9
adrenal glands 97–9
aerobics 45, 47
age factors 7–8, 16–17
alcohol 25, 52
Alexander technique
  40–1
allergies 101–3
androgens 27
antioxidants 90
anxiety 31, 68
aromatherapy 73, 75–6
auto-immune diseases
  18

B

Bach flower remedies
  73, 79

balance, hormones 9,
  16, 72–3, 77
black cohosh 77
body care 50–3
body changes 20–32
bone health 42–4
breasts 24–5, 50–1

C

calcium 86, 98, 108–9
cancer, breast 17–18,
  24–5, 58, 66–7
carbohydrates 42, 88
cardiovascular disease
  29–30
changes 7–10
  body 20–32
  climacteric 15–16
  diet 84–5

self-help 33–4
chiropractic 79
cholesterol 96–7
climacteric 12–16
coffee 85, 87
collagen 26
complementary
  therapies 9, 71–82
continuous combined
  therapy 60
creative imagery see
  visualization
cyclical therapy 59–60

D

depression 31, 65–6, 68
diary-keeping 19–20
diet 9–10, 17–18,
  82–110

E

early menopause 17–18, 29
eating habits 103
elastin 26
emotional symptoms 30–2
endometriosis 67
endometrium, cancer 58
estrogen *see* oestrogen
exercise 41–7, 48, 52–3
eye exercises 52

F

facial exercises 52–3
fats 86–7, 91–4
fertilization 14–15
fibre 90–1
fibroids 67
flexibility 45–6
follicle-stimulating hormone (FSH) 14, 16, 19
follicles 14–16, 19
food issues 83–110
formication 26
friends 35
frown lines 53
fruit 86, 89–90
FSH *see* follicle-stimulating hormone

G

gallstones 67
genetic factors 24, 29, 96–7
genital problems 23
gonadotrophin-releasing hormone (GnRh) 14
gums 27

H

hair 27
Hatha yoga 40
headaches 23–4, 66
heart disease 29–30
herbalism 73, 76–7
homeopathy 73, 78
hormone replacement therapy (HRT) 48–9, 52, 56–68, 73
hormones
    androgens 27
    balance 9, 16, 72–3, 77
    exercise 42
    follicle-stimulating hormone 14, 16, 19
    gonadotrophin-releasing hormone 14
    HRT 48–9, 52, 56–68, 73
    luteinizing hormone 14, 16
    menstrual cycle 13–15
    oestrogen 14–20, 30–1, 57–61, 94–7
    phytoestrogens 94–7
    progesterone 14–16, 58–60
    progestogen 58–60
    stress 97–9
    testosterone 49
hot flushes 22, 36, 69
HRT *see* hormone replacement therapy

hydrotherapy 81, 103
hypothalamus 13–14, 16, 19
hysterectomy 18, 29, 61

I

immune systems 9, 18
implants, HRT 62–3
insomnia 68–9
interests 35–6
intolerances 101–3
isoflavones 95–6

J

jogging 41, 44–6
joint pains 25–6

L

laughter lines 53
LH *see* luteinizing hormone
libido loss 47–9
linseed oil 93
liver disease 67
local treatments 60–1
luteinizing hormone (LH) 14, 16

M

masculinization 27
massage 73, 80–1
meditation 39–40
memory loss 30
menopause 11–20
menstrual cycle 13–15, 18–19
menu plans 85–7
minerals 86, 89–90, 98–9, 104–9

monounsaturated fats 93
mood swings 100–1
mouth 27

N
nails 27
natural therapies 75–82
non-hormonal therapy 61
nutrition 82–110

O
oestrogen
HRT 57–61
menopause 14–20
phytoestrogens 94–7
psychological symptoms 30–1
oils 75–6, 93–4
orthodox treatments 55–70, 72–3
osteopathy 73, 79
osteoporosis 28–9, 41–2, 61, 70
ovaries 14–18, 29

P
patches, HRT 59–60, 62–3
pelvic exercise 48
peri-menopause stage 13
periods 12–15, 17–20
physical symptoms 8, 22–30
phytoestrogens 94–7
pilates 47
pituitary gland 13–14, 16

PMS *see* premenstrual syndrome
polyunsaturated fats 92–3
post-menopause stage 13
power surges *see* hot flushes
pre-menopause stage 12
premenstrual syndrome (PMS) 15, 60, 69–70
progesterone 14–16, 58–60
progestogen 58–60
prolapses 28
prostaglandins 15
proteins 26, 88
psychological symptoms 30–2

R
rebounder 46
recipes 10
see also separate index
refined foods 86
reflexology 73, 80
relaxation techniques 36–41

S
St. John's wort 77
salt 87, 99
saturated fats 91–2
seaweed 98
self-help 8, 33–53
sensitivity, foods 102
sequential therapy *see* cyclical therapy

sex life 8–9, 47–9
side effects 64–6, 71–2
skin 26, 51–2, 106–9
smoking 17, 25, 52, 85
social life 34–6
sodium 87, 99
soya 95–6
stamina 45
sterilization 18
strength 44–5
stress 37, 97–9
strokes 30
supplements 103, 110
symptoms
emotional 30–2
physical 8, 22–30
psychological 30–2
synthetic progesterone *see* progestogen

T
tablets, HRT 59–60, 62–3
tai chi 47
tamoxifen 96
tea 85, 87
testosterone 49
therapies
complementary 9, 71–82
HRT 48–9, 52, 56–68
local 60–1
natural 75–82
non-hormonal 61
orthodox 55–70, 72–3
tibolone 61–3
trans-fatty acids 92
treatments *see* therapies

V

vaginal dryness 70
vegetables 86, 89–90
visualization 38–9
vitamins 89–90, 98–9,
   104–9

W

walking 41, 43–6
water 81, 103
weight 17, 27–8, 66,
   100–1

Y

yoga 40, 47, 73

Recipe index

A

artichokes, chilled
  stuffed artichokes 125

B

baked stuffed
  mushrooms 128
bass with fennel 129
beef 176–9
  beef with broccoli and
    oyster sauce 176–7
  Chinese minced beef
    with tofu 178–9
broccoli and red
  pepper fettuccine
    salad 200–1

C

caponata 196–7

carrot and coriander
  noodle soup 113
carrot and sage soup
  112
chicken 148–67
  chicken with pine
    nuts 156–7
  chicken and prawn
    kebabs 162–3
  chicken with sizzling
    garlic sauce 160–1
  chicken, squash and
    sweet potato tagine
    166–7
  cranberry chicken stir-
    fry with ginger
    148–9
  Malaysian chicken,
    noodle and prawn

stew 214–15
pesto chicken and
  pepper salad 184–5
shredded chicken
  with green peppers
  158–9
Sichuan bang bang
  chicken 150–1
stir-fried chicken with
  cashew nuts and
  baby corn 154
stir-fried chicken with
  pineapple 164–5
Thai green chicken
  curry 155
Thai minced chicken
  with basil 152–3
chilled fresh fruit soup
  115

chilled stuffed
  artichokes 125
Chinese dishes
  braised vegetables
    198–9
  crab soup 119
  minced beef with tofu
    178–9
cod baked with
  potatoes, onions and
  tomatoes 138–9
crab, Chinese crab
  soup 119
cranberry chicken stir-
  fry with ginger 148–9
crispy seaweed 189

D

desserts 216–22
  chilled fresh fruit soup
    115
  melon, grape and
    kiwi salad 222
  melon ice cream 220
  spiced pears 221
  strawberries with
    blackcurrant sauce
    218
  stuffed figs 219
  summer fruit platter
    217
  yogurt-fruit cup 216

F

fish 129–47
  Chinese crab soup
    119
  cod baked with
    potatoes, onions
    and tomatoes

138–9
  fish risotto 212–13
  haddock and fennel
    soup 118
  halibut on a bed of
    vegetables 134–5
  Japanese tofu and fish
    hotpot 132–3
  lobster and corn
    chowder 120–1
  sauté of scallops with
    mangetout 140–1
  sea bass with fennel
    129
  seafood risotto
    210–11
  smoked haddock with
    red pepper sauce
    136–7
  spaghetti marinara
    208
  steamed masala
    mussels 142–3
  steamed spiced fish
    130–1
  stir-fried prawn
    supper 144–5
  stir-fried prawns with
    tofu 146–7

G

green beans with
  broccoli and almonds
  192–3

H

haddock
  haddock and fennel
    soup 118
  smoked haddock with

red pepper sauce
    136–7
halibut on a bed of
  vegetables 134–5

J

Japanese dishes
  miso soup with tofu
    116–17
  seaweed salad 186
  tofu and fish hotpot
    132–3

L

lamb 180–3
  Moroccan lamb
    182–3
  paper-thin lamb with
    garlic and spring
    onions 180–1
lobster and corn
  chowder 120–1

M

Malaysian chicken,
  noodle and prawn
  stew 214–15
melon, grape and kiwi
  salad 222
melon ice cream 220
Moroccan lamb 182–3
mulligatawny soup
  122–3
mushrooms, baked
  stuffed 128
mussels, steamed
  masala mussels 142–3

N

noodles

carrot and coriander noodle soup 113
Malaysian chicken, noodle and prawn stew 214–15

P
paper-thin lamb with garlic and spring onions 180–1
pasta 200-9
  broccoli and red pepper fettuccine salad 200–1
  pasta niçoise 206–7
  spaghetti with anchovies and olives 209
  spaghetti marinara 208
  spaghetti with marinated vegetables 204–5
  tagliatelle with chilli and roast cherry tomato dressing 202–3
  three-bean fusilli salad 188
pesto chicken and pepper salad 184–5
pork 168–75
  pork and vegetables 174–5
  stir-fried pork with tofu and mangetout 170–1
  sweet and sour pork 172–3
  sweet and spicy pork

with pomegranate 168–9
prawns
  chicken and prawn kebabs 162–3
  Malaysian chicken, noodle and prawn stew 214–15
  stir-fried prawn supper 144–5
  stir-fried prawns with tofu 146–7
pumpkin and lemon soup 114

R
raindrop soup 124
rice 210–13
  fish risotto 212–13
  seafood risotto 210–11
roasted beetroot citrus salad 187

S
salads 184–8
  broccoli and red pepper fettuccine salad 200–1
  Japanese seaweed salad 186
  pesto chicken and pepper salad 184–5
  roasted beetroot citrus salad 187
  three-bean fusilli salad 188
scallops, sauté of scallops with mangetout 140–1

seafood see fish
seaweed
  crispy seaweed 189
  Japanese seaweed salad 186
shredded chicken with green peppers 158–9
Sichuan dishes
  bang bang chicken 150–1
  tofu 190–1
smoked haddock with red pepper sauce 136–7
soups 112–24
  carrot and coriander 113
  carrot and sage 112
  chilled fresh fruit 115
  Chinese crab 119
  haddock and fennel 118
  Japanese miso soup with tofu 116–17
  lobster and corn chowder 120–1
  mulligatawny 122–3
  pumpkin and lemon 114
  raindrop 124
spaghetti
  with anchovies and olives 209
  with marinated vegetables 204–5
  spaghetti marinara 208
spiced pears 221
starters 125–8
  see also soups

baked stuffed
  mushrooms 128
chilled stuffed
  artichokes 125
tempura 126–7
steamed dishes
  masala mussels 142–3
  spiced fish 130–1
  vegetables with
    ginger 194
stir-fried dishes
  chicken with cashew
    nuts and baby corn
    154
  chicken with
    pineapple 164–5
  cranberry chicken
    with ginger 148–9
  mixed vegetables 195
  pork with tofu and
    mangetout 170–1
  prawn supper 144–5
  prawns with tofu
    146–7
strawberries with
  blackcurrant sauce
  218
stuffed figs 219
summer fruit platter
  217

sweet and sour pork
  172–3
sweet and spicy pork
  with pomegranate
  168–9

T
tagliatelle with chilli
  and roast cherry
  tomato dressing
  202–3
tempura 126–7
Thai dishes
  green chicken curry
    155
  minced chicken with
    basil 152–3
three-bean fusilli salad
  188
tofu
  Chinese minced beef
    with tofu 178–9
  Japanese miso soup
    with tofu 116–17
  Japanese tofu and fish
    hotpot 132–3
  Sichuan tofu 190–1
  stir-fried pork with
    tofu and mangetout
    170–1

stir-fried prawns with
  tofu 146–7

V
vegetables 189–99
  baked stuffed
    mushrooms 128
  caponata 196–7
  chilled stuffed
    artichokes 125
  Chinese braised
    vegetables 198–9
  crispy seaweed 189
  green beans with
    broccoli and
    almonds 192–3
  pumpkin and lemon
    soup 114
  Sichuan tofu 190–1
  steamed vegetables
    with ginger 194
  stir-fried mixed
    vegetables 195

Y
yogurt-fruit cup 216